Praise for *Long Lever Techniques*

"I write from the perspective of one who experienced the discomfort of coccydynia for many months after a protracted and difficult labor. While that particular discomfort is thankfully now more than four decades in the past, it appears that our understanding of the aetiopathology of coccydynia and the rationale(s) for clinical management of the condition remain 'works in progress'. I therefore have a very personal reason to welcome the blend of anatomy applied to clinical practice and clinical insight that Dr Nourani details in this book."

—SUSAN STANDRING MBE, PhD, DSc, FKC, Hon FRCS,
Emeritus Professor of Anatomy, King's College London,
and Editor-in-Chief of *Gray's Anatomy* (39ed-42ed)

"The Long Lever Technique is a unique blend of principles that were developed by generations of osteopathic pioneers. With a strong basis in anatomy and physics and an understanding of functional physiology (including the primary respiratory mechanism), this technique offers something of value to any of the osteopathic approaches you typically use in your practice."

—RACHEL BROOKS, MD

"A well-organized, efficient, and easy-to-apply treatment that is practical for students, residents, and physicians of all levels."

—MICHAEL A. SEFFINGER, DO

"This is a practical and well-illustrated manual that guides the practitioner through all aspects of applying this technique. I use Long Lever Technique for exaggeration of the lesion in an indirect approach. Now, after reviewing this book I intend to try this more direct method as well."

—ELIOTT BLACKMAN, DO

"Long Lever Technique is a beautiful melding of structure and function and uses the principles of applied anatomy in a direct and efficient manner. It acknowledges the underlying forces of the Breath of Life while addressing the structural problems encountered in both acute and chronic conditions. This book is a welcome addition to the osteopathic literature."

—CHRISTOPHER MULLER

Long Lever Techniques

Long Lever Techniques

An Illustrated Guide
for Practitioners to Treat
Neuro-Musculoskeletal Pain

BOBBY NOURANI, DO, FAAO
RICHARD HUFF, DO

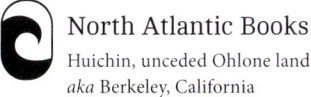

North Atlantic Books
Huichin, unceded Ohlone land
aka Berkeley, California

Copyright © 2022 by Bobby Nourani. All rights reserved. No portion of this book, except for brief review, may be reproduced, stored in a retrieval system, or transmitted in any form or by any means—electronic, mechanical, photocopying, recording, or otherwise—without the written permission of the publisher. For information contact North Atlantic Books.

Illustrations by William Kuchera, Zac Miller, and Bobby Nourani, DO, FAAO

Treatment technique and anatomical overlay photos by Jim Keating

Beauchene skull reprinted with permission from Kenneth Lossing, DO

Historical images reprinted with permission from the Museum of Osteopathic Medicine, Kirksville, MO: [1985.1023.08] Andrew Taylor Still; [2015.67.01] William Garner Sutherland, DO; [1980.482.01] Leather helmet photograph.

Published by   Cover photos by Jim Keating
North Atlantic Books   Cover design by Jasmine Hromjak
Huichin, unceded Ohlone land   Book design by Happenstance Type-O-Rama
aka Berkeley, California

Printed in the United States of America

Long Lever Techniques: An Illustrated Guide for Practitioners to Treat Neuro-Musculoskeletal Pain is sponsored and published by North Atlantic Books, an educational nonprofit based in the unceded Ohlone land Huichin (aka Berkeley, CA), that collaborates with partners to develop cross-cultural perspectives, nurture holistic views of art, science, the humanities, and healing, and seed personal and global transformation by publishing work on the relationship of body, spirit, and nature.

North Atlantic Books' publications are distributed to the US trade and internationally by Penguin Random House Publishers Services. For further information, visit our website at www.northatlantic books.com.

MEDICAL DISCLAIMER: The following information is intended for general information purposes only. Individuals should always see their health care provider before administering any suggestions made in this book. Any application of the material set forth in the following pages is at the reader's discretion and is their sole responsibility.

Library of Congress Cataloging-in-Publication Data

Names: Nourani, Bobby, 1981– author. | Huff, Richard, 1943- author.
Title: Long lever techniques : an illustrated guide for practitioners to
   treat neuro-musculoskeletal pain / Bobby Nourani, DO, FAAO & Richard
   Huff, DO.
Description: First. | Berkeley, California : North Atlantic Books, [2022] |
   Includes bibliographical references and index.
Identifiers: LCCN 2021038713 (print) | LCCN 2021038714 (ebook) | ISBN
   9781623176785 (trade paperback) | ISBN 9781623176792 (ebook)
Subjects: LCSH: Musculoskeletal system—Diseases—Treatment. | Osteopathic
   medicine.
Classification: LCC RC925 .N68 2022 (print) | LCC RC925 (ebook) | DDC
   616.7—dc23/eng/20211008
LC record available at https://lccn.loc.gov/2021038713
LC ebook record available at https://lccn.loc.gov/2021038714

1 2 3 4 5 6 7 8 9 VERSA 26 25 24 23 22

North Atlantic Books is committed to the protection of our environment. We print on recycled paper whenever possible and partner with printers who strive to use environmentally responsible practices.

Dedicated to my family and friends, the best cheerleaders I could have. Dad, your endless love and positive affirmations spring me forward. Mom, your hunger for learning is infectious. My sisters, Moriah and Sereena, your existence alone makes me strive to be a better person. Last but not least, to my mentors and patients who have instilled me with trust and confidence as I have developed. Ultimately this book is dedicated to Dr. Huff, to those he was inspired by, and to those like me who carry on his legacy.

BOBBY NOURANI, DO, FAAO

*In Memory of the Originator of the
Long Lever Technique*

Richard G. Huff, DO

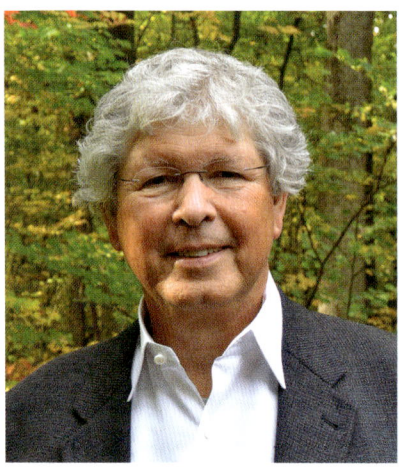

May 7, 1943–January 28, 2019

As members of Dick Huff's family, we watched him build his medical practice, discover new manipulation methods, and develop what ultimately became the Long Lever Techniques outlined in this manual. We often benefited from and were willing participants in his trial-and-error search for improved manipulation. But the professional side of Dick was, in our world, just a part of his wonderful presence. He joined his wife Pat in a grand adventure to build a life they both wanted together. Pat and Dick worked and celebrated together for fifty-one years. He taught his son Brett by example, care, and helpful suggestion. Brett remembers daily Dick's virtues of intellectual curiosity, hard work, empathy, and the joys of a good meal and bottle of wine with family and friends. Later in life, Dick devoted himself to developing relationships with his daughter-in-law and grandchildren. They remember him as a kind soul who pushed them to read books. We can hear his voice in this manual. We know he would be excited to collaborate with so many accomplished physicians, sharing ideas to help improve patient health.

Pat Huff and Brett, Katie, Carter, and Vivian Huff

Dick Huff was deeply accomplished at osteopathic manipulative medicine and an innovative, relentlessly curious physician. He gathered effective but disparate techniques—both those he discovered and developed through experimentation and those he adopted from other expert practitioners—and combined them into a system outlined in *Long Lever Techniques.* I worked closely for many years with Dick at Mercy Health Partners watching and helping him advance and develop the practice of OMM across the United States. But Dick was much more than his professional accomplishments: he was one of my oldest and closest friends. He was kind, caring, humble, empathic, and loving. He loved his wife without condition, was both an exemplary father and a close friend to his son, and loved spending time with his daughter-in-law and his two grandchildren. I hear Dick's ideas and enthusiasm in this manual, and I miss my friend and his smile, tenderness, and wit. I wish all the readers of *Long Lever Techniques* could have known my friend. He was an unparalleled blessing in my life.

Denny Cherette
Former chairman of Mercy Health Partners
Founding member of the Osteopathic Foundation of West Michigan

It was such a privilege for me to know and work with Dick Huff. He was living proof of how fine a person, and a doctor, can be. I can't recall a single time when he was too busy to talk with me or to treat me or a member of my family. A consummate physician and professional in every sense of the word, he was insatiably curious and always open to new techniques and ideas. As a physician and educator, Dr. Huff loved to teach and was loved by those fortunate enough to spend time with him. He had a wonderful smile and twinkling eyes, a sense of humor and a gentle spirit. Dick was incredibly bright, logical, and systematic in his thinking . . . and always willing to share his ideas and information. I so enjoyed my professional relationship with him, but it was truly a treasured gift to be his friend.

Roger Spoelman, DBA, MBA
Former president and CEO of Mercy Health Partners

Contributors

Charlie Beck, DO, FAAO
President, Indiana Academy of Osteopathy
Private Practice
Osteopathic Vision, LLC
Indianapolis, IN

Michael Carnes, DO, FAAO
Associate Professor of Osteopathic Principles
and Practice
University of Pikeville–Kentucky College of
Osteopathic Medicine

Francois L. Cyr, MBA
President, Integrative Management
Services, Inc.
San Diego, CA

Katherine Heineman, DO
Past OMM Department Chair, College of
Osteopathic Medicine, Des Moines University
Private Practice
Osteopathic Care, PLC
Des Moines, IA

Richard G. Huff, DO
Founder and Past Director of Mercy Health
Partners Osteopathic Manipulative Medicine
Clinic
Muskegon, MI

Michael L. Kuchera, DO, FAAO, FNAOME
Secretary-General, Fédération Internationale
de Médecine Manuelle
Professor (retired), OMM/NMM

William A. Kuchera, DO, FAAO, Dist.
Professor Emeritus
Kirksville College of Osteopathic Medicine,
A.T. Still University

Kenneth Lossing, DO
Past President, American Academy of
Osteopathy
Private Practice
San Rafael, CA

Bobby Nourani, DO, FAAO
Private Practice
Lake Forest, CA
Associate Professor, Department of Neuro-
musculoskeletal Medicine/Osteopathic
Manipulative Medicine (NMM/OMM),
College of Osteopathic Medicine of the Pacific,
Western University of Health Sciences
Past Osteopathic Program Director of Clinical
Instruction, University of Wisconsin Depart-
ment of Family Medicine and Community
Health
Past Medical Director of Inpatient Integrative
Health, University of California–Irvine

William P. Powell, DO
Adjunct Clinical Professor, Pacific Northwest
University
Private Practice
Ashland, OR

David Rakel, MD
Esther Millard Professor and Chair, University
of Wisconsin School of Medicine and Public
Health
Department of Family Medicine and Commu-
nity Health

Edward G. Stiles, DO, FAAO, Dist.
Professor, Osteopathic Principles
University of Pikeville–Kentucky College of
Osteopathic Medicine
Director of Neuromusculoskeletal Medicine
Pikeville Medical Center

Benjamin J. Visger, DO
Private Practice
Muskegon, MI
Associate Clinical Professor, Neuromusculo-
skeletal Medicine and Osteopathic Manipula-
tive Medicine
Michigan State University College of Osteo-
pathic Medicine

Contents

PART 3 Coccyx and Craniococcygeal Anatomy

PART 4 Integrating Long Lever Techniques in Practice

Preface

The content and ideas presented here are based on experiences in an osteopathic musculoskeletal medical practice and are intended to be a practical manual. The intention is to put forth a unique and effective treatment technique. The works and teachings from Andrew Taylor Still and William Garner Sutherland provide the foundation for the principles and methods presented in this text. We do not intend to reiterate their thought processes, but rather to advance knowledge or provide a different perspective from which to view these recurring issues in a musculoskeletal practice. The Long Lever Techniques presented in this text combine principles of Osteopathy in the Cranial Field with more manual techniques of the axial skeleton and limbs. The result is time-efficient treatments with good clinical outcomes that can be performed by both novice and advanced providers. We hope this content stimulates clinical growth and applications of osteopathic concepts.

Richard Huff, DO
Bobby Nourani, DO, FAAO

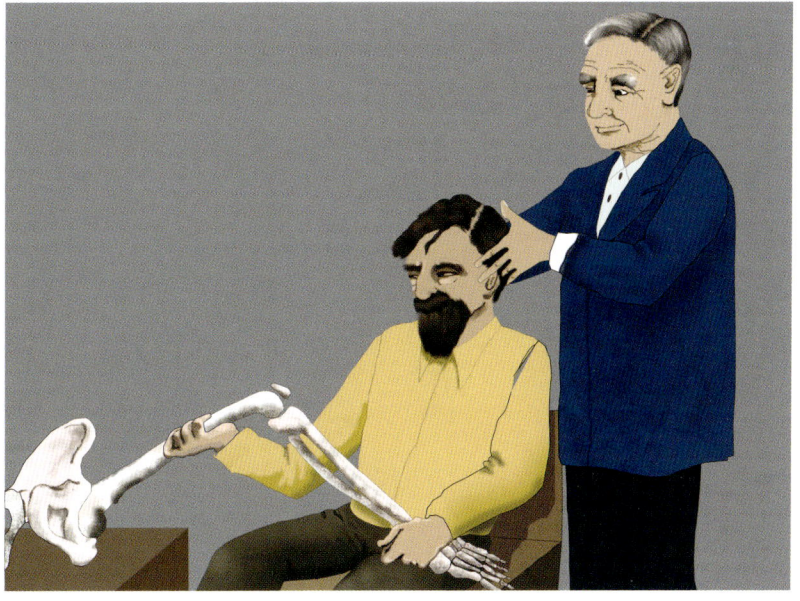

This illustration by Sophia Voelker is recognition of Dr. Huff's inspiration from A.T. Still and W.G. Sutherland.

Foreword

During my Integrative Medicine fellowship at the University of Arizona, part of the curriculum involved going to a variety of different professionals to be a recipient of their art. I received acupuncture, I was given a homeopathic constitutional remedy, and I was hypnotized. But it wasn't until I lay on the table of Harmon Myers, DO, that I was awakened to the potential of how hands, with the right skills, could heal.

Bobby Nourani, DO, joined our Integrative Medicine program at the University of Wisconsin in 2015. He brought with him unique osteopathic skills with an inquisitive mind. But what stood out most was his passion for teaching. He is able to take complexity, simplify it, and make it easy to understand.

Our medical culture is in dire need of change. Addressing complex problems like pain with just one modality resulted in a public health crisis of addiction without better health outcomes. We are in need of a better way that recognizes the unique interplay of the physical body that extends beyond the most painful spot.

The Long Lever Technique does not focus on just one part of the body but demonstrates how we can mobilize distant interconnected structures to positively restore the body to better health and function. The information is taught in a way that physicians and other body workers can learn to put it into practice immediately.

If you are interested in learning how to incorporate osteopathic skills in a busy primary care practice to improve the health of your patients, this book and the technique it describes is a great place to start.

Thank you, Dr. Nourani, Dr. Huff, and your team for providing this valuable resource during a time of great need.

With gratitude,

David Rakel, MD
Esther Millard Professor and Chair
Department of Family Medicine and Community Health
University of Wisconsin School of Medicine and Public Health

Foreword

Bobby Nourani, DO, produces an excellent manual that presents and preserves Richard Huff, DO's approach to osteopathic manipulative treatment (OMT). Paul Kimberly, DO, FAAO, one of the outstanding teachers in the osteopathic profession, stressed "Learn the principles and then get them to work for you." The Long Lever Technique (LLT) is, for me, an illustration of that truth.

Principally, OMT techniques may be classified as follows:

1. *Segmental position* related to the restrictive barrier: direct versus indirect

2. *Corrective force* utilized:

   a. Physician-introduced force, e.g., a thrust or impulse

   b. Patient-introduced force, e.g., a specific muscle effort

   c. Inherent forces, e.g., primary respiratory mechanism (PRM), Mayer waves, or respiration

The key to understanding Dr. Huff's LLT is appreciating that it is a direct approach utilizing inherent forces. The localization to the dysfunctional anatomical layer using a long lever is followed by use of the primary respiratory mechanism to facilitate the correction. The spine or an extremity is utilized as the long lever for localizing the forces at the dysfunctional fascial area. Continuous fine-tuning of the patient's position maintains the dysfunction at the feather's edge of the restrictive barrier to keep the localized layer actively releasing.

I see interesting correlations between Dr. Huff's LLT and the teachings of George A. Laughlin, DO, one of my mentors, and I think the LLT is another application of the basic osteopathic principles. As I watched Dr. Huff treat at the AAO Convocation in 2018, he positioned a patient seated for treatment similarly to how Dr. Laughlin positioned patients. Specifically, Dr. Laughlin taught that if spinal translation is utilized in three planes while the patient is in the sitting position, one activates Fryette's third principle and turns the patient's spine into a long lever. Laughlin's approach could be viewed as an indirect long lever technique.

Dr. Huff's use of the LLT is a novel description and approach synthesized from the traditional osteopathic principles.

Ed Stiles, DO, FAAO, Dist.

Professor, Osteopathic Principles

University of Pikeville–Kentucky College of Osteopathic Medicine

Director of Neuromusculoskeletal Medicine

Pikeville Medical Center

Foreword

The co-authors and contributors successfully present a great deal of value in *Long Lever Techniques*. More than offering technique alone, the text contains thought-provoking observations and pearls of insight that, in combination, present a unified approach to managing health and function.

Richard Huff, DO: I knew Dr. Huff from a patient care and research network dedicated to management of patients with gravitational strain pathophysiology and sagittal plane postural decompensation. Our approach integrated individualized prescriptions for orthotics, osteopathic manipulative treatment (OMT), and exercise. To optimize patient health, our network of physicians sought long-lasting, global responses from neuromusculoskeletal tissues, visceral function, and primary and secondary respiration. Dr. Huff would not only identify the key precipitating factors bringing patients to his office, he sought and initiated solutions to perpetuating factors. I believe that the *long-lasting* results from the *Long Lever* Techniques delineated in this book are an extension of his *long-term* philosophy to address perpetuating issues.

One strength of this manual is the inclusion of Dr. Huff's detailed "History and Progression of the Long Lever Technique." It should provide insight for those with diverse educational backgrounds by delineating component elements that he integrated from different teachers, along with his interpretation.

Bobby Nourani, DO, FAAO: Despite being fellows of the same academy (the American Academy of Osteopathy), Dr. Nourani and I did not know each other well until we shared a long flight together coming back from an AAO Convocation. Our "lofty" discussions at 35,000 feet promoted ongoing and profound (and sometimes lofty) osteopathic dialogues that I hope he values as much as I do! I find great satisfaction in having an insightful colleague with whom to debate nuanced issues that might otherwise be more accurately shared kinesthetically.

Dr. Nourani and his invited contributors obviously worked hard to overcome some of the limitations imposed by traditional biomechanical nomenclature (as defined in the *Glossary of Osteopathic Terminology*[1]) to describe the unique contribution of LLT and its

---

[1] Giusti, R. (Ed.). (2017). *Glossary of osteopathic terminology* (3rd ed.). Chevy Chase, MD: American Association of Colleges of Osteopathic Medicine.

xxii   *Long Lever Techniques*

application to the treatment of a patient with somatic dysfunction. In this regard, I do have a few observations to share that may be useful. For example:

◆ Classification of OMT in this manual: Thinking locally, on face value one might see the setups described in the manual for these techniques as "direct method techniques," and I have no doubt that locally there are direct actions taking place on the tissues responsible for local somatic dysfunction barriers. But as Drs. Huff and Nourani uniquely add, LLT techniques specifically monitor primary respiratory mechanism characteristics in the area and continuously adjust the long lever forces to maintain an inherent force focus at the feather's edge of dynamically changing pseudo-barriers. This is reminiscent of several master practitioners whose techniques (including BLT/LAS) often combine direct and indirect methods into the integrated technique. Using Kimberly's OMT taxonomy, I would probably classify the techniques in this manual as representative of a "combined method with inherent force activation." (Again, read Dr. Huff's "History and Progression." Ed Stiles's "Foreword," which Dr. Nourani wisely included, presents his perspective as well.)

◆ Designation of the purported somatic dysfunction: Somatic dysfunction is defined as "impaired or altered function of related components of the somatic (body framework) system: skeletal, arthrodial, and myofascial structures and related vascular, lymphatic, and neural elements." Traditional reporting of spinal somatic dysfunction focuses on naming the dysfunction for its pattern of asymmetrical motion characteristics; this, in part, because OMT using local or short lever strategies to correct the somatic dysfunction typically localizes forces at a vertebral unit or a vertebral unit component (such as a facet). By convention, vertebral units are named for the superior of the two vertebrae involved. Interestingly, depending on your palpation method (active or passive) as well as the layer or structures being assessed, different diagnoses with different motion characteristics might result. Here the manual's discussion by Charlie Beck, DO, FAAO, "The Quantum of Healing: Interexaminer Reliability," should be strongly considered. It may also be helpful to some readers to note that in our discussions, Dr. Nourani notes that, for thoracolumbar spinal diagnoses, he and Dr. Huff similarly used a combination of "hardness" over a transverse process, followed by the dynamic effect locally from active flexion and extension by the patient. (In my experience, this best identifies facet motion characteristics and often helps determine direct muscle energy setup for thoracic or lumbar FRS or ERS somatic dysfunctions.)

Throughout this manual, Dr. Nourani largely holds to traditional osteopathic naming conventions (including use of Fryette and other osteopathic designations from the *Glossary*) to delineate where the local somatic dysfunction was identified and what its conventional diagnosis might be. (Naming vertebral unit somatic dysfunction for the top segment and/or the effect of its inferior facet are internally consistent with traditional thoughts for performing spinal OMT.) Although this convention works exceedingly well in understanding short lever techniques and the initial setup depicted in the manual for top-down LLT techniques, it can be confusing when discussing bottom-up LLT.[2] It might be helpful to consider that by its multifactorial nature and various tissues involved, LLT affect and are affected by much more than just one vertebral unit.

Nonetheless, seeking LLT resolution of pseudo-barriers and ultimately true barrier somatic dysfunction is not dependent on spinal mechanics alone. In the techniques described in this manual, I found it very useful to review Dr. Huff's historical description of his diagnostic criteria—namely, the subsection emphasizing the "Concept of Hardness." Regardless of your diagnostic approach or any traditional Fryette-style thoracic or lumbar designation, the somatic dysfunction being treated using this LLT approach is determined by the location of the "hardness." The initial biomechanical setup is guided by your diagnostic palpations and considerations of how that vertebra is affected in its motion with the rest of the body.

Many physical therapy or manual medicine texts include nonspecific long lever techniques; and, until now, few osteopathic technique manuals have detailed specific long lever techniques. *Long Lever Techniques* is long overdue and greatly expands the osteopathic discussion of specific long lever versus short lever techniques. It additionally contributes to the relatively sparse literature on treatment approaches that could be used to affect the sacrococcygeal joint (and adjacent ganglion impar) while also providing an application of the LLT in a way that I have not seen before.

Uniquely, clearly, and concisely, this manual describes "combined method with inherent force activation" OMT techniques designed to help practitioners leverage longer-lasting resolution of somatic dysfunction and systemic integration of local function.

Michael L. Kuchera, DO, FAAO, FNAOME

Secretary-General, Fédération Internationale de Médecine Manuelle

Professor (retired), OMM/NMM

---

[2] For the extremities, diagnostic nomenclature can be adjusted to reflect bottom-up or top-down dysfunctions. For example, the relative positions and motion characteristics are the same for "posterior glide of the talotibial joint" and "anterior glide of the tibiotalar joint" somatic dysfunctions. The choice of which diagnostic terminology is preferred is often made after deciding on treatment and whether the talus or the tibia is addressed relative to the other. By convention, vertebral unit dysfunction is always named from the top down, and this presents a logistical challenge in linking it to bottom-up LLT techniques. In this manual, for example, hand placement and pseudo-barrier monitoring for a purported T10 somatic dysfunction are described as focusing on T9 and T10 (which would traditionally define the T9 vertebral unit); likewise, in this manual, L3 and L4 are contacted to address a purported L4 somatic dysfunction from the bottom up. Discarding strict use of segmental thoracolumbar designations better recognizes that motion/function of a single vertebra can be affected by multiple somatic influences from both above and below. So again, the reader is referred to Dr. Huff's diagnostics and treatment for the use of LLT at a given site regardless of what the designation is for the segmental (vertebral unit) component.

PART 1

Development of
Long Lever Techniques

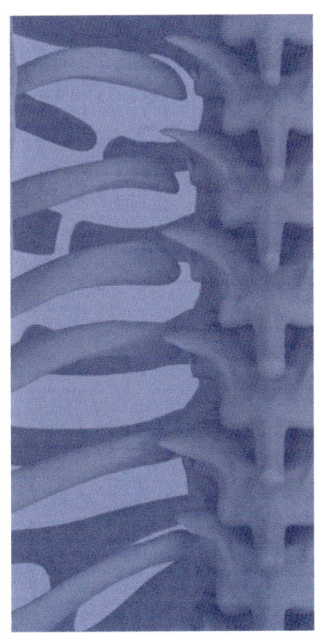
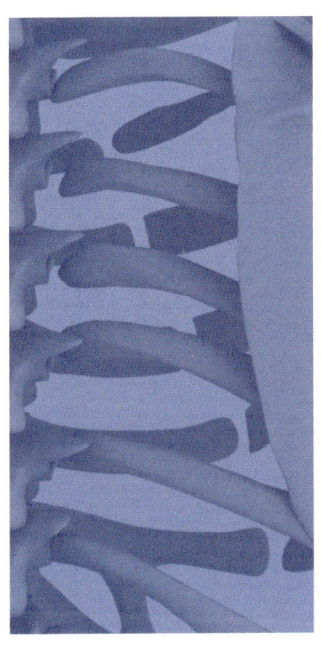
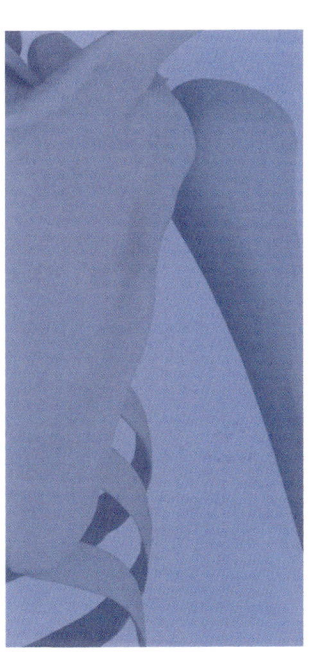

Introduction

BOBBY NOURANI, DO, FAAO

This book introduces an osteopathic manual medicine treatment approach not yet documented. Long Lever Technique is a direct treatment to normalize flow of the primary respiratory mechanism at the site of somatic dysfunction. Immediate benefits include reestablishing the cranial rhythmic impulse (CRI), primary respiratory mechanism (PRM), and/or inherent potency at the site of dysfunction. It is a direct treatment technique improving the PRM of restricted skeletal structures by applying concepts of Osteopathy in the Cranial Field to the axial skeletal system. Integrating proper structural mechanics of the spine with the PRM produces profound effects. This direct technique improves tolerability for the elderly patient, without the audible "pop" inherent with high-velocity, low-amplitude (HVLA) techniques. Compared to Muscle Energy Technique, requiring active patient involvement, LLT is a passive and practitioner-driven technique. Patient positioning and treatment are adjusted according to the PRM. The site of the somatic dysfunction demarcates interruption of the PRM quality and amplitude proximal and distal to the affected site. Use of the appendages and head as long levers creates an amplified input flow of the PRM directed to the fulcrum that is the area of somatic dysfunction. This provides a greater output flow of the PRM released through the restricted barrier. Long-lasting benefits include increased mechanical range of motion and ultimately enhanced and normalized PRM potency of the affected skeletal structures. Identifying the areas of greatest restriction and normalizing the primary respiratory mechanism across the restriction reduce the number of areas requiring treatment.

Original credit for education of Long Lever Techniques is respectfully due to the teachings and wisdom of Richard Huff, DO. Dr. Huff was a graduate of the A.T. Still University, Kirksville class of 1970. In 2007 I first witnessed Dr. Huff's creative treatment approach that yielded a high-quality benefit in a relatively short treatment duration. Through his direct teaching and my own clinical experience with patient improvement, I became convinced that other clinicians would appreciate this knowledge as well.

My Osteopathic History

RICHARD HUFF, DO

Long Lever Technique arose from many years of clinical practice trying to understand and apply a variety of disparate osteopathic concepts. It has taken years of practice to learn to evaluate a patient, identify where and how to begin treatment, and then apply treatment with osteopathic manipulation to completion. The results of this effort are presented in *Long Lever Techniques* with the hope of making the reader's journey easier and more productive in the management of common medical problems.

Growing Up in Kirksville

I regarded the well-known practice of osteopathy from an early age, as nearly all local practitioners in Kirksville were osteopathic physicians. By the late 1950s and early 1960s, Missouri had fully licensed osteopathic physicians, and at that time most osteopaths practiced general or family care. Many performed some form of osteopathic manipulative treatment (OMT), mostly high-velocity, low-amplitude (HVLA) techniques, directed at the area of complaint and largely based on Dr. Andrew Taylor Still's teaching of "find it, fix it, and leave it alone." Regardless, I was too young at the time as a teenager to truly understand the core concepts of osteopathy.

Although none of my family members were physicians, I nonetheless had many positive interactions with osteopathy that guided me to this as my life's work. I frequently interacted with osteopathic students and physicians when my grandparents took in boarders from the school. Occasionally, my grandparents would board well-known osteopaths such as Dr. Benjamin Jolly, whose history with then-named Kirksville College of Osteopathic Medicine (KCOM) has been prominently displayed in one of the academic halls at the school. It was during this integral time that Dr. Jolly facilitated my early interest in general practice. While I was an osteopathic medical student, he helped me secure weekend work at a hospital where he worked in Moberly, Missouri.

I also entertained osteopathic ideas through interactions with friends who went on to be osteopathic physicians. One friend since middle school, Patrick Laughlin, DO, deserves special mention. His father, George Laughlin, DO, operated one of the few osteopathic practices in town that focused primarily on OMT. I learned about the teaching of Dr. William Garner Sutherland, whose theories eventually formed some of the basis of Long Lever Techniques, as he had formally trained under the elder Dr. Laughlin. I had many positive connections with prominent osteopathic physicians throughout my middle and high school years, including Dr. Kim Korr, Dr. David Korr, Dr. Elliott Hix, and Professor Claus Rohweder, DO. It even led me to participate in osteopathic research, as I was one of many research subjects for Dr. J. S. Denslow, a professor and respected osteopathic researcher. This invaluable exposure to notable osteopathic greats and their families contributed to my love of osteopathy.

Not all of my interactions with osteopathy as a young man were positive, however. One particularly negative experience was with an osteopathic physician to whom my mother referred me for low back pain. This physician treated me with a lumbar roll HVLA technique that unfortunately exacerbated my pain so much that I became stooped over and unable to attend a school dance that evening. Additionally, when I became a physician, my wife was generally hesitant to receive high-velocity treatments for neck pain due to her personal beliefs and fears. I feel fortunate these negative experiences did not dampen my enthusiasm for osteopathy, but instead motivated me to seek and practice alternative OMT techniques that ultimately resulted in the development of the Long Lever Techniques.

Early Years at KCOM

Three significant events ultimately contributed to developing Long Lever Techniques. First, I became a KCOM neuroanatomy fellow and studied under Olwen Gutensohn, DO, and her successor, Donald Vedral, PhD, DO, who taught the neuroanatomy course at KCOM. I took the fellowship in part because it was a way to enact Dr. Still's call to "dig on." The fellowship was one attempt to reach the "next layer" of understanding to benefit the patient. This fellowship provided training in neuroanatomical dissection, initiating my interest in cranial OMT, and provided my first insight into academic medicine, which, while compelling, solidified my preference for clinical osteopathic work.

Second, Herbert Miller, DO, became an instructor at KCOM and introduced the then-emerging Osteopathy in the Cranial Field as a course of study to interested students at KCOM, which was fully supported by Dr. Sutherland. As part of this course, I met with and observed treatments performed by eminent cranial manipulators, including Herbert Miller, DO; Robert Fulford, DO; Harold Magoun, DO; Alan Becker, DO; and Rollin Becker, DO. I was very interested in this approach, given my negative experience with HVLA. At a Sutherland Cranial Academy meeting, I watched the prominent osteopaths present and discuss this emerging manipulative option. I learned about the primary respiratory mechanism (PRM) and cranial motion but had yet to feel them myself. These concepts provided the foundation for what ultimately became Long Lever Techniques, though, at the time, I was unaware of their significance and influence in developing my practice and methods.

Third, I met the incoming KCOM Osteopathic Manipulative Medicine (OMM) Chairman Keith Buzzell, DO, who eventually became an important mentor, with whom I became acquainted because of James Jealous, DO, the KCOM anatomy fellow at that time. I was fortunate to have met so many exemplary physicians and researchers, as noted, during my time at KCOM and have benefited greatly from each of these mentors. I proudly share these experiences to encourage students to seek out mentors during their training.

Understanding the Importance of the PRM and Cranial Motion

My understanding of the importance of the PRM and cranial motion developed over time, though a few milestones are worthy of note. Although I initially did not understand or feel the PRM, I came to accept that I should, and would, be able to accomplish this skill. In my clinical practice, I set aside time every day with one patient to explore this concept.

I first attended a Sutherland Cranial Teaching Foundation (SCTF) course in 1967, where sufficient compelling evidence and discussion helped me embrace the concept of cranial bone motion. When I listened to the SCTF instructors and other practitioners at the conference, there appeared to be unanimity and consensus in regard to cranial bone motion. The conversations about cranial bone motion were complex due to the nuanced nature of the phenomenon. The majority of my classmates dismissed this as "mystical," but I was open to the idea, as I trusted Drs. Still's and Sutherland's theories were grounded in anatomy and physiology. Therefore, I focused my efforts in these two disciplines, but with a variation in the clinical application of treatment.

Consequent to my wife's refusal to allow HVLA treatment of her neck, I did not use many HVLA techniques in my own practice. It became clear early on that HVLA techniques were not going to be as useful as I had been led to believe in medical school. After all, if my wife refused to let me "crack her neck," even when indicated, where was I supposed to go from there?

At this time there were many visiting lecturers to KCOM who presented newly developing OMM concepts. Osteopathic innovation had accelerated, and the lecturers were a remarkable window into these new ideas. Fortunately, Dr. Jealous and I had joined in many informal discussions with visiting lecturers on their thoughts and practice during our fellowship year. During this time, a number of new osteopathic techniques were being developed in the field, and I was privy to these new vistas and gained valuable perspective.

As a result of all of this, I began a more serious study and practice of the cranial concept. By this time, I could palpate cranial motion, but I was still unsure if I was feeling the phenomenon the early cranial experts felt. Due to my desire to understand the cranial concept, I applied its principles as often as possible in treating patients, friends, family—including myself. Early on, I made little progress improving patient function when using cranial motion and would then often resort to more familiar OMT methods.

Opportunities for Clinical Focus

Completing my education, I felt fortunate to have had rich training experiences, partake in discussions with eminent and innovative osteopaths, and become more specialized with an introduction to neuroanatomy and cranial motion. I had yet to crystallize my experience and early ideas into a more concrete theory and practice to increase patient benefit. Though the right ingredients to develop the Long Lever Techniques existed for me—exposure to new ideas, a focus on cranial motion, a desire for an alternative to HVLA, encouraging mentors, and a willingness for trial-and-error experimentation—I was still far from a more complete OMT methodology.

Fortunately, I saw two opportunities as I initiated my clinical practice. First, many of the osteopathic innovations at the time had yet to be systematized into a more traditional "peeling the onion" methodology characterized by more traditional osteopathic practice. Second, I saw that the osteopathic canon had yet to embrace, fully, the concept of cranial motion and PRM. As my early private practice evolved, I focused on these two "white spaces" in osteopathic practice.

Starting Clinical Practice

Like many physicians, I struggled to choose my first clinical location. As my education neared its conclusion, I was using osteopathic manipulation routinely, but in a more rote manner. Additionally, I had developed an interest in neurology because of my neuroanatomy fellowship. Both of my options were compelling: attend the only osteopathic neurology residency in the United States or join two KCOM friends and start an emergency room practice at Muskegon General Hospital. Although I was intrigued by the neurology residency in Detroit, Michigan, I decided against it out of worry for my family's quality of life in Detroit as I worked long hours, and due to recent riots occurring in the city. I gratefully joined the new ER practice, and developed a general/family practice with my colleagues at the end of my internship.

After six years of ER practice, I grew tired of the "nights and fights" typical of ERs, and the routine of primary care, leading to two significant changes in my career path. First, I happily accepted the position as medical director in a newly opened Michigan state prison. Second, I redefined my primary care private practice to focus solely on musculo-skeletal medicine.

Simultaneously, a nearby orthopedic surgeon had begun to refer patients to me for sports, workplace, and auto-accident-related problems because of my increasing expertise in OMT. Even more important, I began to see better patient outcomes using a broader variety of OMT techniques while using the PRM and cranial motion. I had taken a number of continuing medical education classes and was using a variety of osteopathic manipulative methods in my family practice. I was starting to see improvement in patients with musculo-skeletal problems in my office practice, which motivated me to perform more OMT in the prison as well. Managing the chronic medical, social, and legal complexities of prisoners' lives is not typically associated with average patient populations. I was encouraged that the more complex prison patient population responded positively to my evolving OMT skills. Once again, I felt I was making progress with systematizing more common osteopathic techniques and incorporating Osteopathy in the Cranial Field.

While patient outcomes progressed, there were other challenges. I started to notice that some patient populations—such as heavily muscled, obese, or just large patients—did not respond to techniques I was taught in school. These challenges provided the impetus, once again, to study more to improve my skills in OMM. Although I had at this point developed a method to localize forces, the technique failed in these populations because effective localization using HVLA was just difficult. I also determined that some patients had poor somatic awareness, making Muscle Energy Technique inefficient, as it required substantial cooperation to localize the forces. Additionally, although I had gained a feel for Osteopathy in the Cranial Field, it was of limited use in my busy practice because of its time-intensive nature. The increasing number of patients seeking my care indicated I was succeeding at some level; but despite my success with patients, it was taking a significant toll on my own physical health and stamina. I was tired and my hands were sore. I was challenged with wanting to provide a high quality of care for my patients, increase daily patient volumes, and develop my manual skills further. Once again, I needed to create and innovate a sustainable and effective method of treatment. Enter the Long Lever Technique.

History and Progression of the Long Lever Technique

RICHARD HUFF, DO

Experimenting with Techniques

I built my practice based mostly on Muscle Energy Technique and had integrated imaging (mostly X-rays), lifts, orthotics (based on teachings of Robert Irvin, DO), and allopathic medicine. I also had a solid referral base, which, to me, validated some of my newer treatment approaches. However, while I continued seeking new treatment modalities, I still found patients who did not respond to the variety of techniques I was using.

I considered a variety of techniques. I believe high-velocity, low-amplitude (HVLA) is a useful osteopathic technique and can successfully reset the nervous system; however, I find a number of limitations to HVLA. For one, localization is difficult to attain, as many patients "tense up" in anticipation of the force they know is coming, the HVLA "pop." In my review of post-treatment findings, the hallmark HVLA "pop" does little to change dysfunction; rather, it seems to move surrounding hypermobile segments. I was also uncomfortable using HVLA in elderly or osteoporotic patients because of the significant forces used.

I explored Strain-Counterstrain Technique. This differs from Long Lever Technique in that it is a purely muscular technique; it does not typically utilize the primary respiratory mechanism (PRM). I ultimately determined that tapping into the PRM was an important factor for better outcomes.

I found Indirect Osteopathic Technique to be difficult. As a practitioner primarily oriented to direct techniques, I could not determine when I had reached an end point and often perceived the motion as going through recurring loops without resolution.

As noted, I also explored and heavily relied on Muscle Energy Technique; it matched my direct-technique preference. It has the one major drawback that lack of somatic awareness in some patients makes initiating muscular effort difficult and results in poor localization. Patients who provide too little or too much effort make maintaining the barrier difficult and time consuming. Some are unable or unwilling to provide enough effort to produce movement of somatic dysfunction, and it can take time to achieve doctor-patient correlation of forces.

After trying various modalities, I determined that I needed to use the PRM, both peripherally in the limbs and centrally in the cranium and spine. I identified the PRM as the ideal source to facilitate therapeutic processes. However, I had yet to consistently harness, direct, or focus this source.

Concept of Hardness

Using hardness to identify somatic dysfunction is quicker and more effective for me than more traditional tissue texture changes, asymmetry, restricted motion, and tenderness (TART). The use of TART has limitations as well, including challenging inter-rater reliability, difficulty identifying the primary dysfunction, and possible lengthy time to find the abnormality.

I suggest the following principles to identify and treat the hardest area:

1. Patient history helps determine a good starting point.

2. Screen a large area using palpation to find the hardest area, and treat it first.

3. Inquire about etiologies of other areas of hardness found upon screening, such as long-forgotten injuries, accidents, or trauma.

4. Use multiple positions: seated, standing, lying down, or the position in which the complaint is exacerbated.

5. Keep the palm at a 90-degree angle to the assessment area to provide the most reliable and repeatable results; the operator can palpate the spinous processes and avoid surrounding muscular or fatty tissues that may give confusing information.

6. Use the palm of the hand to quickly move from the initial area to areas of the spine above and below.

7. Touch the area the patient presents even if it is not the hardest, to help assure the patient their concern was heard, but still treat the hardest area first.

8. Acknowledge painful areas indicated by the patient, but pain/tenderness is not as reliable an indicator as hardness to find the key treatment area.

9. "Peel the onion" using the above steps repeatedly until hardness is resolved.

Utilizing Long Lever Techniques (LLT)

It is important to recognize the two forces that are utilized in the LLT: operator forces and inherent forces. Operator forces are those applied through a long lever, such as an upper or lower extremity. Inherent forces will be discussed later. Both forces are critical to the success of the LLT.

With the patient properly positioned, use the long lever to apply a direct technique using the appropriate extremity or other long lever as shown in the technique visuals. This enables the practitioner to localize forces at the barrier. This barrier is a dynamic, rather than static, barrier, so forces must be continually applied at the *feather's edge* of the somatic dysfunction until there is a release.

Using the Long Lever Technique, the physician can localize the forces at the barrier without any patient input. The longest levers on a patient are the extremities, and they allow the practitioner to appropriately localize all forces and save operator energy. Once the operator's forces are localized at the barrier, the expansion/contraction of the inherent forces of the PRM start to improve the motion of the somatic dysfunction. The application of these two forces, the operator levering through the patient, and inherent expansion and contraction of the PRM, are the key to utilizing the Long Lever Technique.

Somatic dysfunctions at the lumbar level and inferior are more commonly treated using the lower extremity as the long lever. Somatic dysfunctions above the lumbar are more commonly treated using the upper extremity as the long lever. Typically, if treating a lumbar somatic dysfunction, the practitioner's forces are applied from below the dysfunctional segment using one of the lower extremities. One finger contacts the area of dysfunction, while another finger contacts the segment above to monitor and maintain localization. For example, using the lower extremity, the practitioner applies force to the barrier at the L4 spinous process, with an additional finger positioned on the L3 spinous process to monitor. In some cases, when the treatment is not successful, the forces can be applied opposite the more common approach using an upper extremity to apply the operator's forces. Somatic dysfunction at L4 would be localized to that segment while the practitioner then palpates the spinous process at L5 to assure the forces do not go past the L4 barrier.

As the dysfunction begins to improve, the practitioner persistently reengages this dynamic barrier by taking up the slack produced by the expansion/contraction of the inherent forces. The practitioner's forces must be maintained at the feather's edge to get the best results. Being at the feather's edge, as described by early osteopathic physicians, means localizing all the planes of force (flexion/extension, sidebending, rotation, and compression/traction) at the point where the dysfunction begins to be in the most restricted state. It takes time, skill, and understanding before the feather's edge concept can best be put to use. The technique visuals show the proper starting positions. The force planes are then localized by increasing flexion/extension, adduction/abduction, and rotation to the balance tension point, or the feather's edge, of the dysfunctional barrier. The operator then continually engages this barrier as it moves. Patients often complain of pain or will tense up if the practitioner localizes the lever past the barrier. Conversely, it is important not to underengage the barrier, which happens when practitioners fail to engage all planes of the barrier.

The initial steps of the Long Lever Technique involve direct operator forces via a lever localized to the feather's edge of the barrier, which then directs the inherent therapeutic forces of the PRM toward the barrier. The next step is to detect the normal movement of the somatic dysfunction being treated. The final barrier has been treated when the PRM is observed locally and in the immediate surrounding structures. For example, L4 will start to move into flexion/extension as it begins to normalize. The practitioner is looking for a full or reasonably uninhibited range of motion of L4 in all planes before assisting the patient back to a more neutral position. Experience will help determine this normal range of movement. When treatment is complete, the segment may move freely in all planes and be minimally inhibited, lighter, healthier, or just not as hard.

Initially, I thought this freeing to be the end of the treatment. Unfortunately, patients often did not maintain improvement. I came to the conclusion that an additional aspect of the treatment process should be considered: integration.

Integration is a term often bandied about in OMT discussions, and so it should be understood from the standpoint of LLT. For our purposes, it is when the segment comes into sync with its environment. For example, L4 integration means the L4 segment along with the vertebrae above and below all move into flexion/extension, etc., together. Ideally, all lumbar vertebrae should move in synchrony with the PRM once integrated. The thinking is that once integration occurs, the treated structure is more likely to maintain correction when in tune with its surroundings. This integration separates pseudo-barriers from the final restrictive barrier (more to come on that later). When the final restrictive barrier is treated and integrated, the PRM can then be detected at the original dysfunction site and throughout surrounding structures.

After performing a treatment, it is important to support the patient slowly back into a neutral position. This reduces voluntary muscle firing, allowing treated structures to continue to return to homeostasis, and does not reintroduce pain when in a relatively vulnerable position, as is the setup for a direct treatment. This should be done for the first 20–30 degrees out of the treatment position.

At this point, if the practitioner believes the primary dysfunction has been successfully treated, the patient is asked for their perception of pain and improvement. If other important areas of hardness are identified, those areas should be treated before the patient is questioned.

Extended Touch

The practitioner can also use what I call "extended touch" to assess the peripheral areas, such as the thoracolumbar junction, the sacrum, or other myofascial structures. Extending touch is very much like driving a car. One holds the steering wheel; and while turning it, even though you have no direct contact with the wheel, you are very much in control of the motion. This allows for palpation of surrounding structures beyond the anatomical points directly beneath the practitioner's fingers. Using this extended touch allows the practitioner to determine whether peripheral areas need to be treated. Additionally, extended touch includes layered palpation. Once the dysfunctional segment is engaged utilizing LLT, the practitioner may also find it helpful to extend their touch to other potential restricted layers, e.g., muscle, fascia, bone, ligament, nerve, etc.

Summary: Applying the Long Lever Technique

1. Obtain the patient history: primarily the chief complaint localized to the symptomatic area.
2. Screen for hardness: identify the hardest site as the initial area for treatment. Make an osteopathic diagnosis.
3. Position the patient at the dynamic barrier using LLT principles.
4. Apply direct operator forces to the dynamic barrier, treating all pseudo- and final barriers.
5. Obtain motion using the inherent forces of the PRM.
6. Integrate the segment or anatomical area.
7. Question the patient as to improvement.
8. Move on to the next-hardest area.
9. Treat until patient's symptoms improve and/or PRM is reintegrated through all areas.

Questions, Troubleshooting, and Discussion

Reasons for failure of the technique may include not localizing the operator's forces properly, making an incorrect diagnosis, or applying too much operator force, creating patient discomfort. An indication of too much operator force is muscle tensing, or movement of the patient trying to escape the operator's excessive force. Because the operator's forces are so attuned to the barrier, caution should be used in the amount of force applied. Encourage the patient to speak if there is too much discomfort. How does the practitioner know if the technique has failed? This would be indicated by the lack of freedom of motion after three or four cycles of expansion/contraction of the inherent forces.

When patients are questioned regarding improvement, it is important to listen closely to their responses. If the patient states that the pain is still present, you should clarify if the pain is sharp versus achy. Persistent, sharp pain indicates lack of improvement in the somatic dysfunction causing their symptoms. This is due often to either an incorrect diagnosis or an improperly applied technique. Reassess the patient. If the patient states the pain as achy, it is most likely persistence of inflammation. This should subside within 24–48 hours with rest, increased water intake, or a mild analgesic.

At times, patients will notice little to no improvement. Through palpation, the practitioner should notice improvements in motion, fluid flow, or myofascial tenseness. It may be necessary to adopt a wait-and-see approach. Reschedule the patient to see how they are doing later. It is not uncommon for osteopathic treatment to take a few days to reach full improvement. In patients with poor somatic awareness or other impediments to improvement, this may help determine how to proceed.

As we have discussed, not all patients respond to osteopathic manipulative treatment. Some reasons could include:

1. The area treated was not the most significant for their problem.

2. The osteopathic modality applied was not tolerated by the patient.

3. The osteopathic technique was incorrectly applied.

4. The patient's problem was primarily biochemical or psycho-emotional rather than anatomical.

It is important to approach each encounter with the belief that the patient wants to improve. It is common in patients to think that nothing is wrong, based on previous exams. The history or physical exam during your pretreatment evaluation will show important issues to potentially be addressed for patient improvement. The patient's response to treatment may serve as a guide to how long you treat them. If there is no improvement after three treatments, it is unlikely that osteopathic manipulative treatment, at least in my experience, will be effective. In chronic cases, if there is steady, even slow, improvement, it is worth continuing to see the patient for a reasonable period of time. The question is how long is that period of time. A reasonable time period should be three to six months. General guidelines to follow are:

1. Get the acute problem resolved in one to three treatment sessions.

2. Decide whether the practitioner can benefit the patient with the problem.

3. Resolve the chronic problem and discharge from care, or achieve maintenance status in which the patient is seen every one to six months to ensure continued progress.

In complicated problems, it is helpful to have a methodical approach bringing additional resources to bear such as:

1. Devising a treatment plan.

2. Screening the entire body for additional areas of hardness, if not already accomplished.

3. Extending touch to surrounding areas to see if there are areas of hardness/ dysfunction that persist.

4. Utilizing an appropriate exercise program.

5. Utilizing appropriate prescription or over-the-counter medication.

6. Ordering laboratory testing or imaging as needed.

Two things happen early in practice that I would suggest the practitioner guard against. The first is treating patients over and over for the same problem without improvement. Early in my practice, I just knew I could get every patient to improve if I tried harder. As I discussed, some things just don't improve, for whatever reason. The best advice is to talk with the patient about their lack of progress and discharge them so they can try to find someone who can help them. This allows you to move on to patients you can help, as well as allowing the patient to find other options for treatment. Second, seeing patients who have failed all previous treatment does not necessarily mean they cannot improve. A thorough history and physical examination may reveal a treatable problem that has been missed.

The importance of weeding out patients who are not progressing, and being able to bring in new and interesting patients, keeps your practice fresh and keeps you engaged.

Treating the Barrier

BOBBY NOURANI, DO, FAAO

A barrier is often dynamic, meaning it can shift or change. As described by Dr. Huff, dynamic barriers include a true or final barrier and may additionally include one or more pseudo-barriers. Unlike the treatment of a pseudo-barrier, treatment of a true barrier results in integration of the primary respiratory mechanism of the dysfunctional segment with its surrounding structures.

Normal Range of Motion

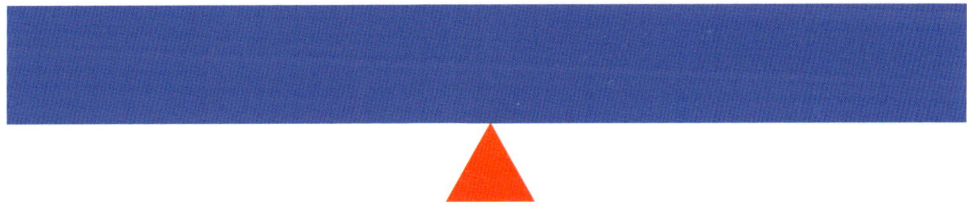

Pseudo-Barrier vs. (True or Final Barrier)

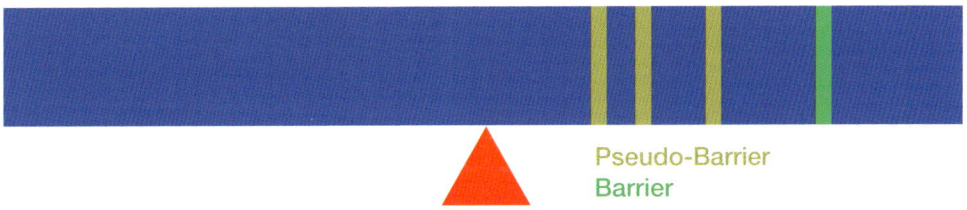

Pseudo-Barrier
Barrier

Potential indications of successful treatment include:

1. Palpation of flexion/extension or internal/external rotation for single or paired bones, respectively.

2. Area of restriction no longer feels hard.

3. Area feels lighter.

4. Nerve roots are no longer restricted.

5. Pain may turn achy. Commonly, patients feel sharp pain with palpation at the areas of dysfunction prior to treatment. With successful treatment, this turns to an achy sensation due to the remaining time it takes for dissipation of cytokines, edema, etc.

Explanation of Long Lever Technique

BOBBY NOURANI, DO, FAAO

This technique is applied to the localized structure(s) of greatest restriction. The structure of greatest restriction may include any of the following: bone, fascia, dura, peripheral nerve, perineurium, muscle fiber, tendon, etc.

This is a direct technique requiring the practitioner to engage the edge of the barrier. Constant adjustments of the long lever are needed to maintain the feather's edge of the barrier. These adjustments may include pressure, angulation, flexion, extension, sidebending, rotation, compression, and traction. Fine-tuning and precise adjustments of the long lever allow for a faster therapeutic response.

Understanding the Concept of a Lever

In terms of physics, a lever is a rigid bar with a handle that pivots on a fixed point to transmit force. The fixed point is often called a fulcrum. If a fulcrum has two sides, one would be considered the side allowing an input force, and the other side would allow for an output force. The amplification of input force to output force is respective of the location

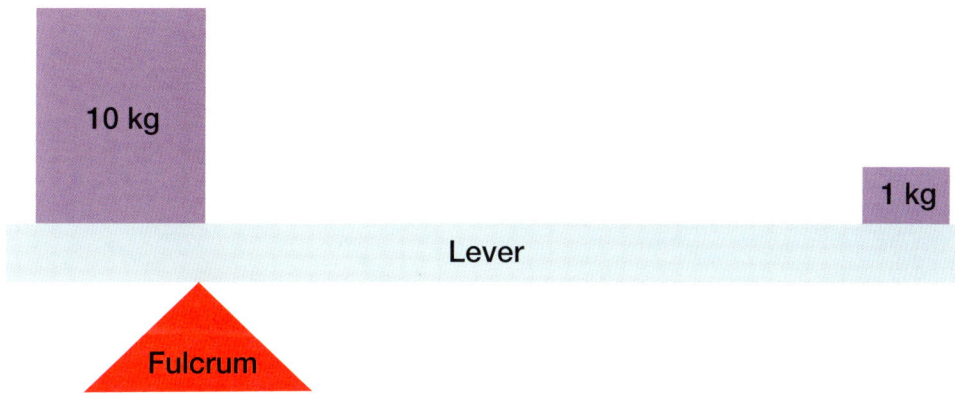

of the fulcrum yielding a mechanical advantage. In the example below, the lever allows for an exertion of a large force over a small distance on one end of the fulcrum, balanced by a small force over a large distance on the other side of the fulcrum. When treating, the longer the lever used, the less input force is needed by the practitioner.

Key Points

1. Use the longest lever possible (i.e., if treating the lumbar, use the foot rather than the knee).

2. Constantly fine-tune and adjust, to stay at the feather's edge of the barrier.

3. If the patient starts to tense up, likely too much force is being applied by the practitioner. To avoid this, keep a placatory awareness at the site of somatic dysfunction and the fulcrum. Slightly engage the barrier, allowing the PRM to reintegrate and release through the barrier. If excessive physical force is applied, the PRM will not reintegrate.

How to Choose Whether to Apply a Long Lever from Above or Below the Site of Dysfunction

The direction of application is based on the direction of impact. Treat from above if the dysfunction feels like it came from above. This can be guided by clinical history. For impacts from above, the long lever is commonly the head, neck, or upper extremity. The restricted superior segment will be engaged by the long lever while the practitioner stabilizes the segment directly inferior.

Treat from below if the dysfunction feels like it came from below. The lower extremities will commonly be used as long levers. The restricted inferior segment will be engaged by the long lever while the practitioner stabilizes the segment directly superior.

> Note: The above is a generality. There may be episodes in which the impact comes from above the dysfunction, but treatment may require access of a long lever from below.

PART 2

Clinical Applications of Long Lever Techniques

BOBBY NOURANI, DO, FAAO

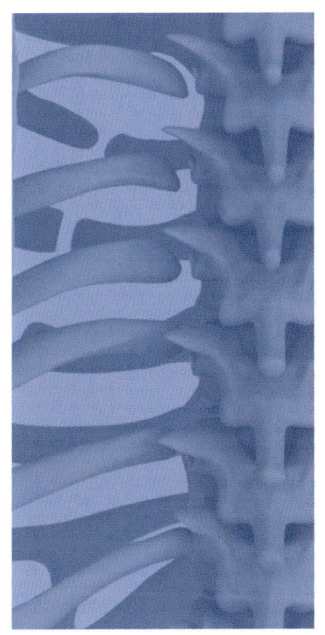
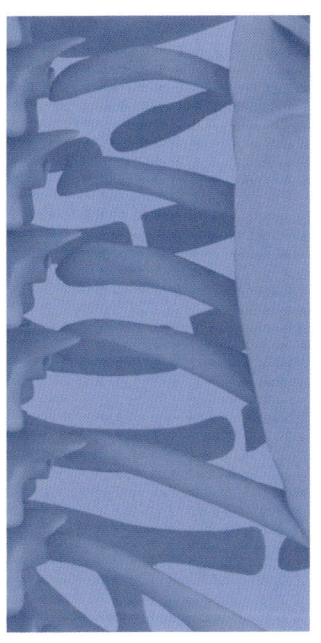
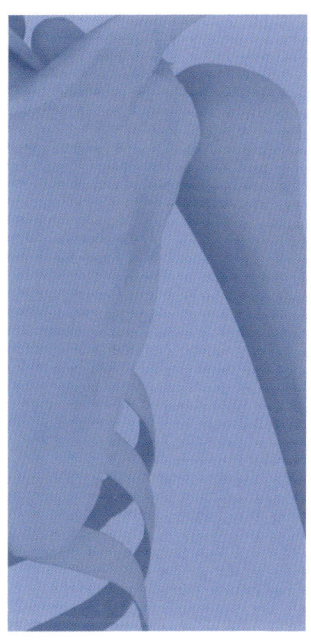

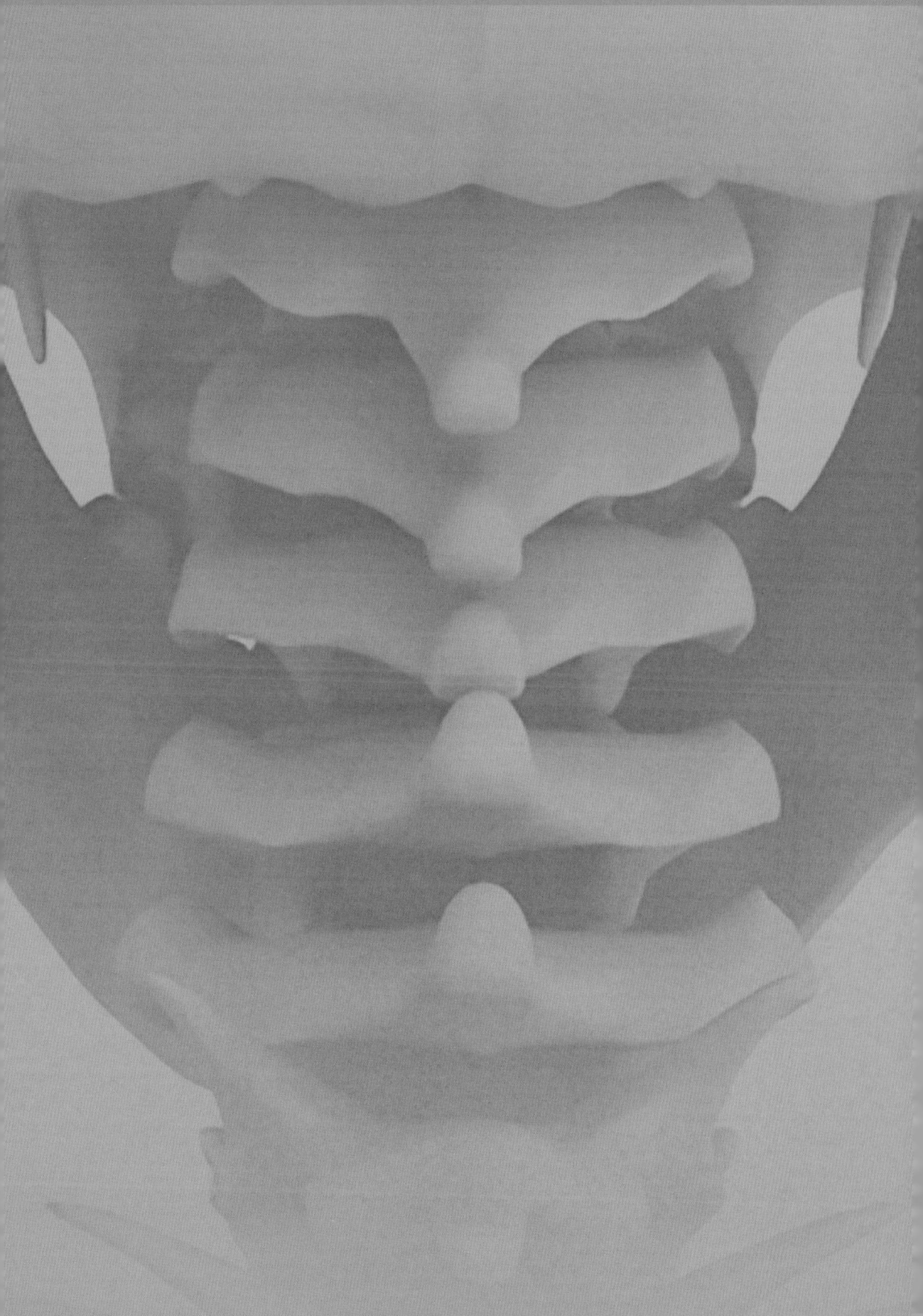

CERVICAL

Diagnosis: C4ERS_R (Extended, Rotated and Sidebent Right)

Treatment position: C4FRS_L (Flexed, Rotated and Sidebent Left)

- ◆ Patient position: Supine. For demonstration purposes, the hand positioning in the photos were taken with the patient seated, but the ideal treatment position is supine.

- ◆ Long lever: Patient's head.

- ◆ Left finger of operator firmly stabilizes neutral vertebra (C5) at the left transverse process or articular pillar. Treatment positioning primarily targets rotation.

- ◆ Engage the barrier: Using the patient's head, introduce flexion and rotation left at the dysfunctional vertebra (C4). Enhance by monitoring at the neutral vertebra (C5).

- ◆ Treatment is complete when the dysfunctional vertebra (C4) has moved through all pseudo-barriers and the final barrier. This is followed by palpation of the PRM at the level of the dysfunction (C4) coordinated with surrounding vertebrae (C3 and C5).

- ◆ Conclusion: Ease the patient out of the engaged position, providing support back to neutral. Releasing the first 15 degrees back to neutral should be done slowly to avoid retriggering the somatic dysfunction.

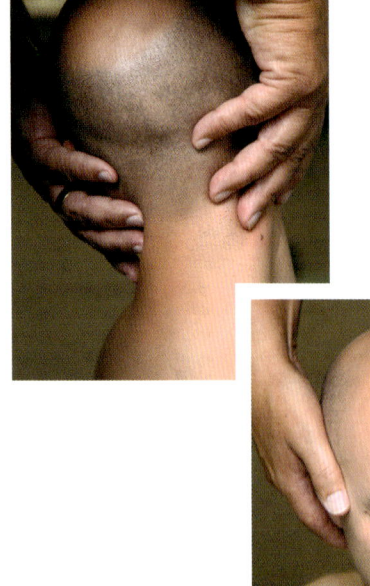

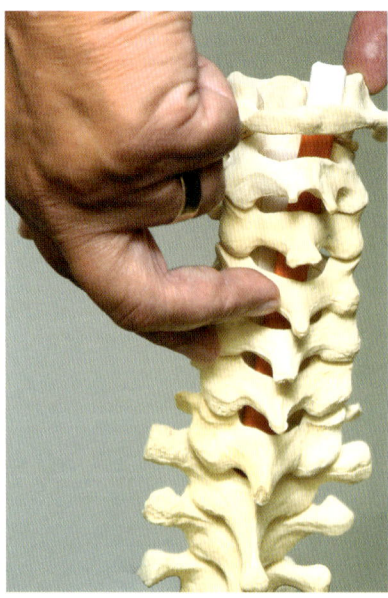

Diagnosis: C4FRS$_R$ (Flexed, Rotated and Sidebent Right)

Treatment position: C4ERS$_L$ (Extended, Rotated and Sidebent Left)

- ◆ Patient position: Supine.

- ◆ Long lever: Patient's head.

- ◆ Left finger of operator firmly stabilizes neutral vertebra (C5) at the left transverse process or articular pillar. This creates a fulcrum to localize extension at the dysfunctional vertebra (C4). Treatment positioning primarily targets rotation.

- ◆ Engage the barrier: Using the patient's head, introduce extension and rotation left specifically at the dysfunctional vertebra (C4). Enhance this by monitoring at the neutral vertebra (C5).

- ◆ Treatment is complete when the dysfunctional vertebra (C4) has moved through all pseudo-barriers and the final barrier. This is followed by palpation of the PRM at the level of the dysfunction (C4) coordinated with surrounding vertebrae (C3 and C5).

- ◆ Conclusion: Ease the patient out of the engaged position, providing support back to neutral. Releasing the first 15 degrees back to neutral should be done slowly to avoid retriggering the somatic dysfunction.

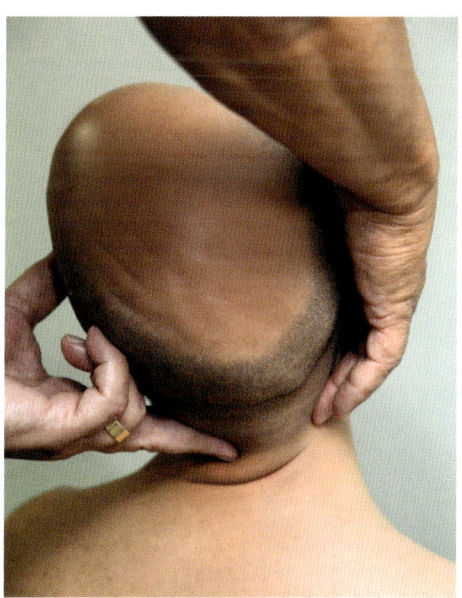
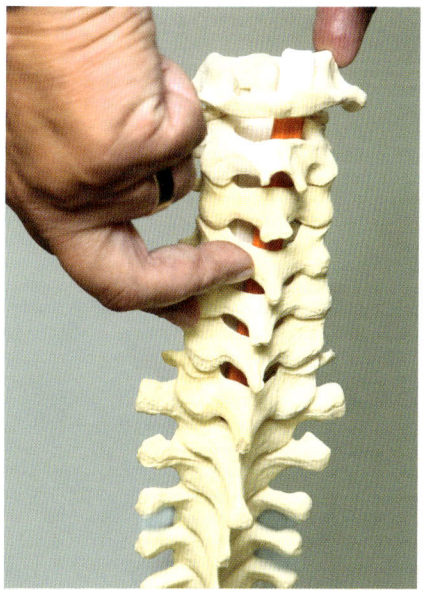

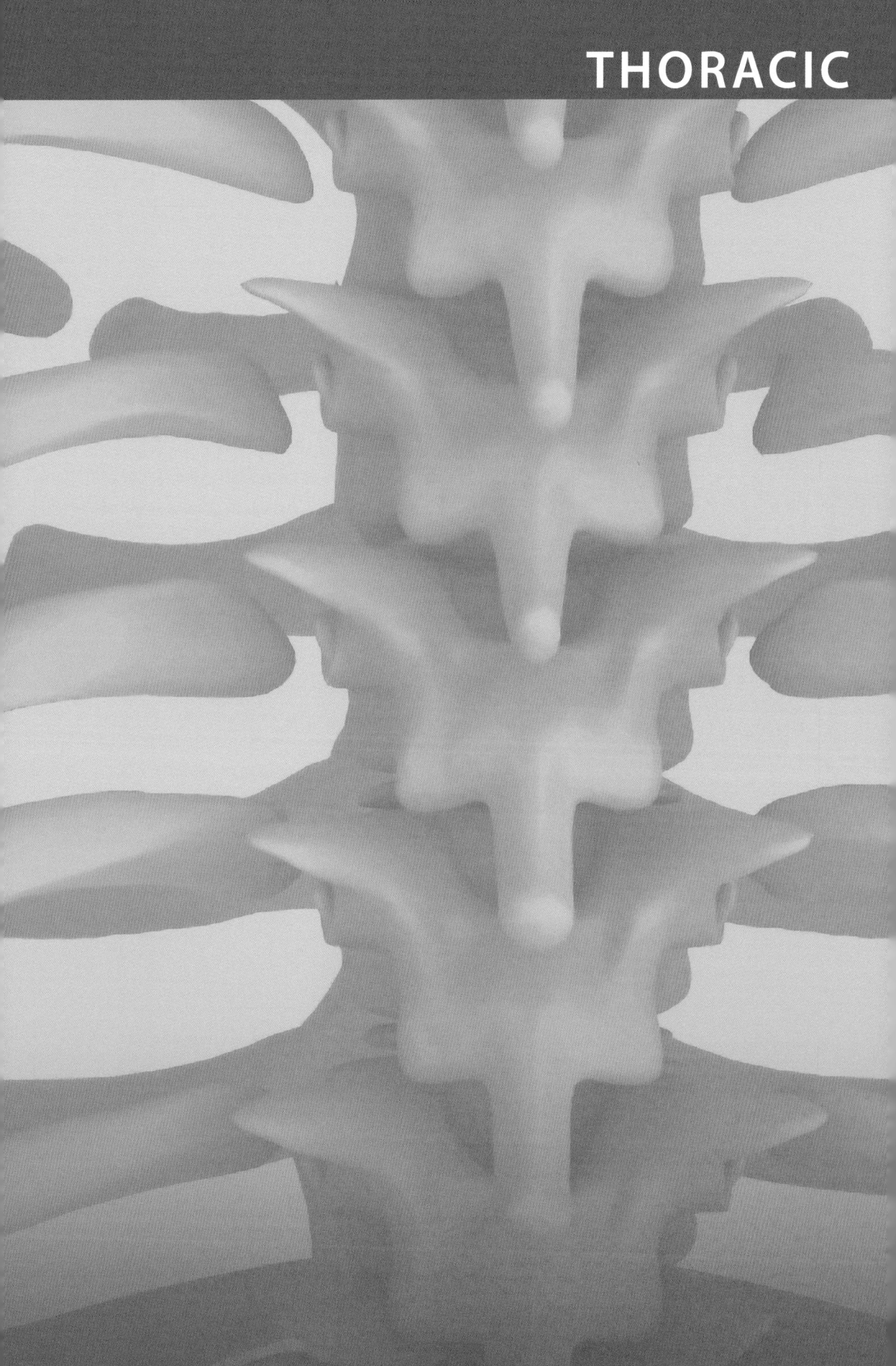

Diagnosis: T2ERS*L* (Extended, Rotated and Sidebent Left)

Treatment position: T2FRS*R* (Flexed, Rotated and Sidebent Right)

- ◆ Patient position: Seated.

- ◆ Long lever: Patient's head.

- ◆ Middle finger monitors and stabilizes left transverse or spinous process (ipsilateral to side of diagnosis) of neutral vertebra (T3) for entire setup and treatment. Index finger monitors the dysfunctional vertebra (T2) at the posterior (left) transverse process.

- ◆ Engage the barrier: Using the patient's head, flex, sidebend right, and rotate right specifically to the dysfunctional vertebra (T2). This is enhanced by monitoring at the neutral vertebra (T3).

- ◆ Treatment is complete when the dysfunctional vertebra (T2) has moved through all pseudo-barriers and the final barrier. This is followed by palpation of the PRM at the level of the dysfunction (T2) coordinated with surrounding vertebrae (T1 and T3).

- ◆ Conclusion: Ease the patient out of the engaged position, providing support back to neutral. Releasing the first 15 degrees back to neutral should be done slowly to avoid retriggering the somatic dysfunction.

> *Note: There are times when the operator may find it necessary to change the side of the upper extremity used for the long lever to better localize to the area of somatic dysfunction. In other words, the direction of positioning would be the same, but the side of the long lever would be opposite.*

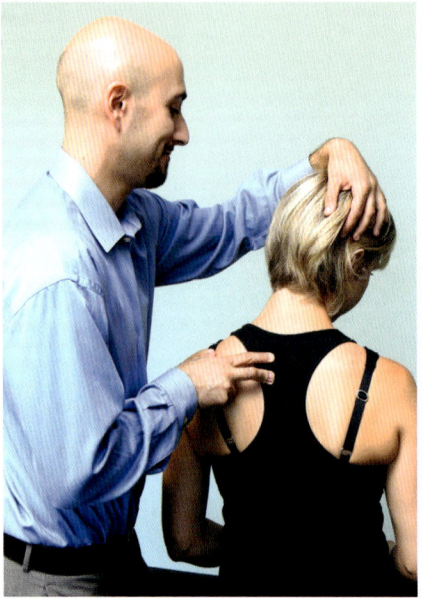
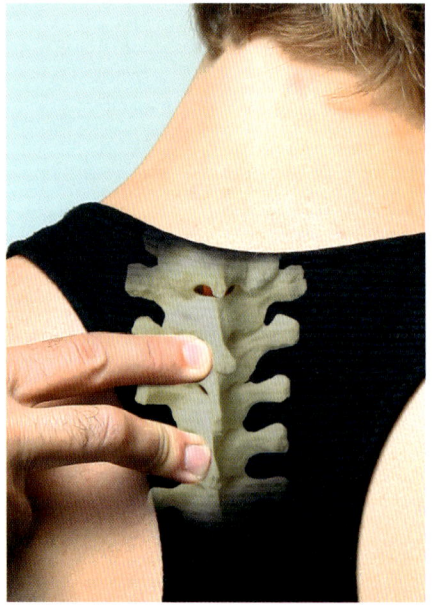

UPPER THORACIC

Diagnosis: T2FRS$_L$ (Flexed, Rotated and Sidebent Left)

Treatment position: T2ERS$_R$ (Extended, Rotated and Sidebent Right)

- Patient position: Seated.

- Long lever: Patient's head.

- Middle finger firmly stabilizes the left transverse process (ipsilateral to side of diagnosis) of neutral vertebra (T3). This creates a fulcrum for localization of extension at the dysfunctional vertebra (T2). Index finger monitors the dysfunctional vertebra (T2) at the posterior (left) transverse process.

- Engage the barrier: Using the patient's head, extend, sidebend right, and rotate right specifically at the dysfunctional vertebra (T2). This is enhanced by monitoring at the neutral vertebra (T3).

- Treatment is complete when the dysfunctional vertebra (T2) has moved through all pseudo-barriers and the final barrier. This is followed by palpation of the PRM at the level of the dysfunction (T2) coordinated with surrounding vertebrae (T1 and T3).

- Conclusion: Ease the patient out of the engaged position, providing support back to neutral. Releasing the first 15 degrees back to neutral should be done slowly to avoid retriggering the somatic dysfunction.

Note: There are times when the operator may find it necessary to change the side of the upper extremity used for the long lever to better localize to the area of somatic dysfunction. In other words, the direction of positioning would be the same, but the side of the long lever would be opposite.

UPPER THORACIC

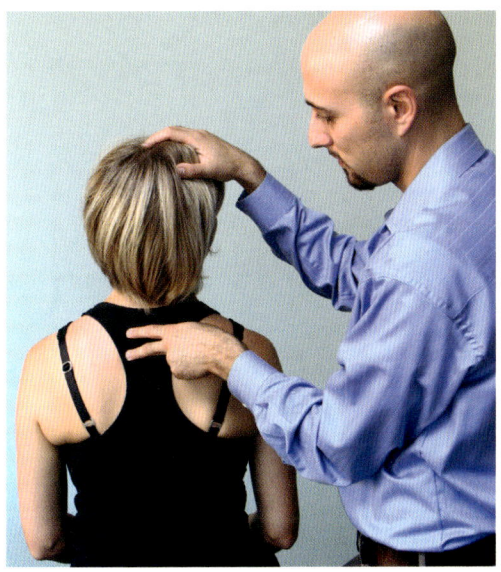
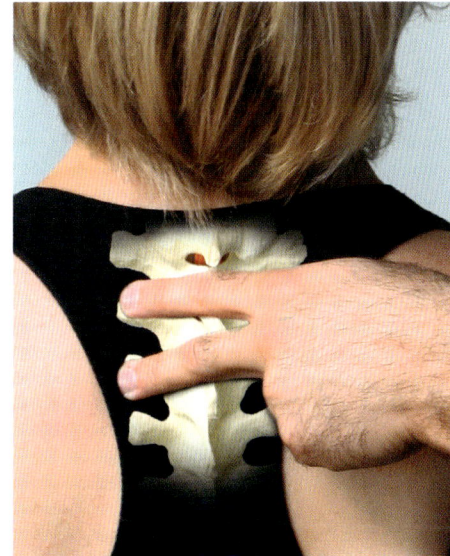

Diagnosis: T7ERS$_L$ (Extended, Rotated and Sidebent Left)

Treatment position: T7FRS$_R$ (Flexed, Rotated and Sidebent Right)

- ◆ Patient position: Seated. Legs extended straight forward with heels on table to stabilize pelvis and lower extremities.

- ◆ Operator stands opposite (right) to the side of diagnosis.

- ◆ Long lever: Left shoulder (ipsilateral to side of diagnosis).

- ◆ Middle finger monitors and stabilizes the neutral vertebra (T8) at the left transverse process (ipsilateral to side of diagnosis). Index finger monitors the dysfunctional vertebra (T7) at the posterior (left) transverse process.

- ◆ Engage the barrier: Using the patient's shoulders, flex, rotate right, and sidebend right specifically at the dysfunctional vertebra (T7). This is enhanced by monitoring at the neutral vertebra (T8).

- ◆ Treatment is complete when the dysfunctional vertebra (T7) has moved through all pseudo-barriers and the final barrier. This is followed by palpation of the PRM at the level of the dysfunction (T7) coordinated with surrounding vertebrae (T6 and T8).

- ◆ Conclusion: Ease the patient out of the engaged position, providing support back to neutral. Releasing the first 15 degrees back to neutral should be done slowly to avoid retriggering the somatic dysfunction.

Note: There are occasions when it is necessary, for better localization, to change the side of the upper extremity used for the long lever. In other words, the direction of positioning would be the same, but the side of the long lever would be opposite.

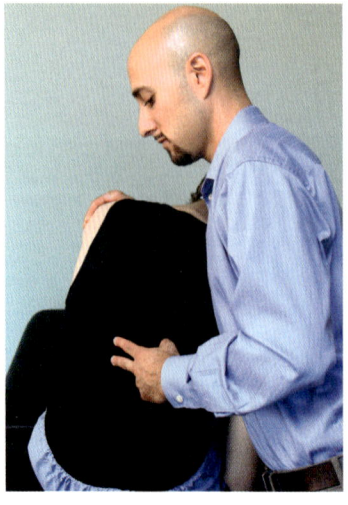
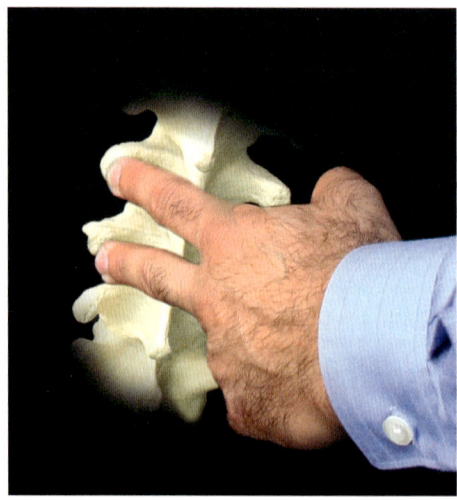

MIDDLE THORACIC

Diagnosis: T7FRS$_L$ (Flexed, Rotated and Sidebent Left)

Treatment position: T7ERS$_R$ (Extended, Rotated and Sidebent Right)

- Patient position: Seated. Legs extended straight forward with heels on table. This stabilizes the pelvis and lower extremities.

- Operator stands opposite (right) to the side of diagnosis.

- Long lever: Left upper extremity with contact at the elbow (ipsilateral to side of diagnosis).

- Middle finger firmly stabilizes the neutral vertebra (T8) at the left transverse process (ipsilateral to side of diagnosis). This creates a fulcrum for localization of extension at the dysfunctional vertebra (T7). Index finger monitors the dysfunctional vertebra (T7) at the posterior (left) transverse process.

- Engage the barrier: Using the patient's left upper extremity (ipsilateral to side of diagnosis), extend, rotate right, and sidebend right at the dysfunctional vertebra (T7). This is enhanced by monitoring the neutral vertebra (T8).

- Treatment is complete when the dysfunctional vertebra (T7) has moved through all pseudo-barriers and the final barrier. This is followed by palpation of the PRM at the level of the dysfunction (T7) coordinated with surrounding vertebrae (T6 and T8).

- Conclusion: Ease the patient out of the engaged position, providing support back to neutral. Releasing the first 15 degrees back to neutral should be done slowly to avoid retriggering the somatic dysfunction.

Note: There are occasions when it is necessary, for better localization, to change the side of the upper extremity used for the long lever. In other words, the direction of positioning would be the same, but the side of the long lever would be opposite.

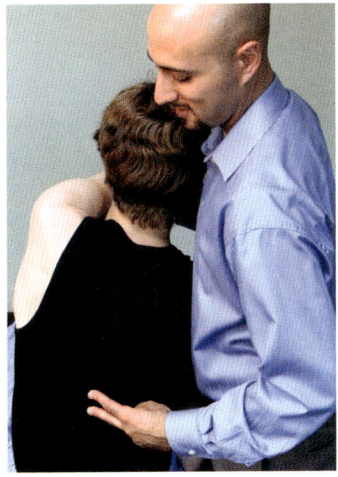
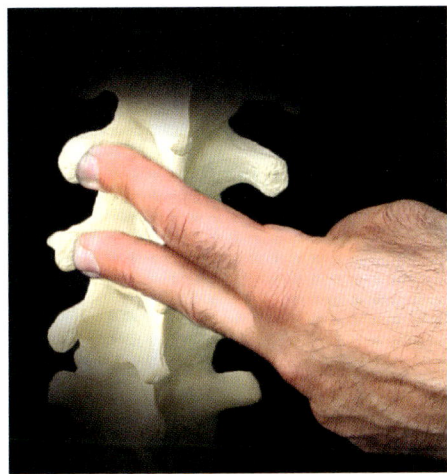

Diagnosis: T10ERS$_L$ (Extended, Rotated and Sidebent Left)

Treatment position: T10FRS$_R$ (Flexed, Rotated and Sidebent Right)

- Patient position: Prone.

- Index finger monitors right transverse or spinous process (contralateral to side of diagnosis) of vertebra above (T9) for entire setup and treatment.

- Engage the barrier: Flex and abduct the right lower extremity (contralateral to side of diagnosis) at the hip with knee bent approximately 90 degrees. This induces right rotation of the dysfunctional vertebra (T10) relative to the above vertebra (T9). With the patient's left knee bent, operator abducts the left hip until motion is localized to engage the dysfunctional vertebra (T10) relative to the above vertebra (T9).

- Long lever: Left lower extremity (ipsilateral to side of diagnosis). Internally rotate the hip by taking the foot laterally and cephalad to lock out the barrier. This uses two planes of motion to localize the barrier more accurately. Maintain appropriate pressure at the right transverse process of the neutral vertebra (T9) to prevent it from rotating right.

- Treatment is complete when the dysfunctional vertebra (T10) has moved through all pseudo-barriers and the final barrier. This is followed by palpation of the PRM at the level of the dysfunction (T10) coordinated with surrounding vertebrae (T9 and T11).

- Conclusion: Ease the patient out of the engaged position, providing support back to neutral. Releasing the first 15 degrees back to neutral should be done slowly to avoid retriggering the somatic dysfunction.

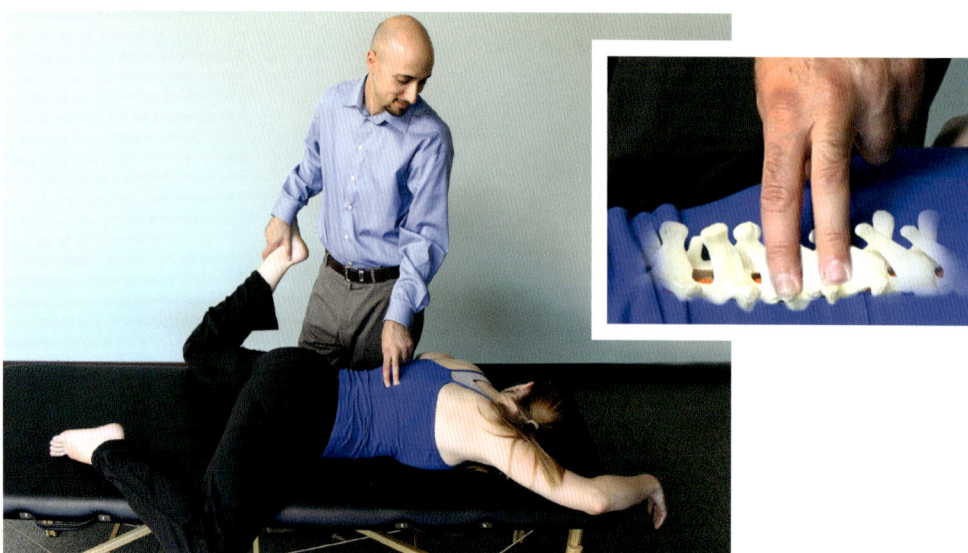

Diagnosis: *T10FRS$_L$ (Flexed, Rotated and Sidebent Left)*

Treatment position: T10ERS$_R$ (Extended, Rotated and Sidebent Right)

- Patient position: Prone, on elbows to induce extension from above (i.e., prone prop position). Induce right thoracic sidebending (contralateral to side of diagnosis) by drawing both lower extremities laterally to the right.

- Monitor at right transverse processes (contralateral to side of diagnosis) of the above vertebra (T9) and the dysfunctional vertebra (T10) for entire setup and treatment. Firmly stabilize right transverse or spinous process of T9 to prevent right rotation.

- Long lever: Extended right lower extremity (contralateral to side of diagnosis).

- Engage the barrier: Support right lower extremity (contralateral to side of diagnosis) proximal to the knee. Introduce extension at the hip to the dysfunctional vertebra (T10). Adduct and externally rotate the right lower extremity to engage right rotation of the dysfunctional vertebra (T10).

- Treatment is complete when the dysfunctional vertebra (T10) has moved through all pseudo-barriers and the final barrier. This is followed by palpation of the PRM at the level of the dysfunction (T10) coordinated with surrounding vertebrae (T9 and T11).

- Conclusion: Ease the patient out of the engaged position, providing support back to neutral. Releasing the first 15 degrees back to neutral should be done slowly to avoid retriggering the somatic dysfunction.

Note: If having difficulty locking out the right lower extremity (contralateral to side of diagnosis), consider inducing further external rotation by weighing down the right knee or adding a pillow under the right foot.

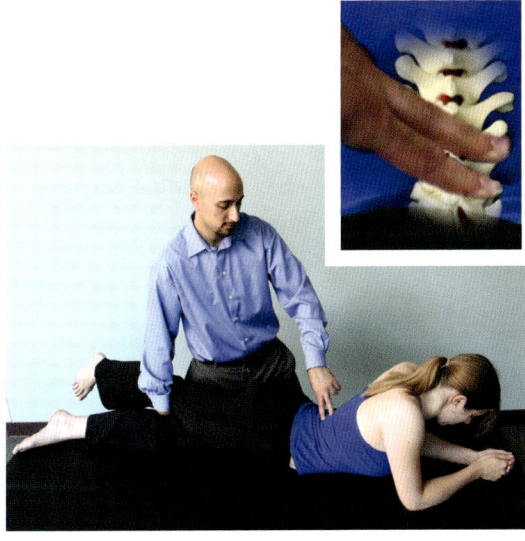 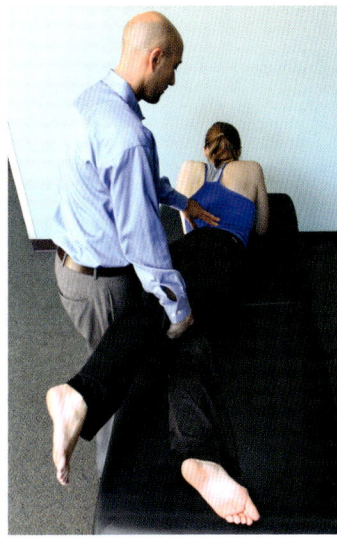

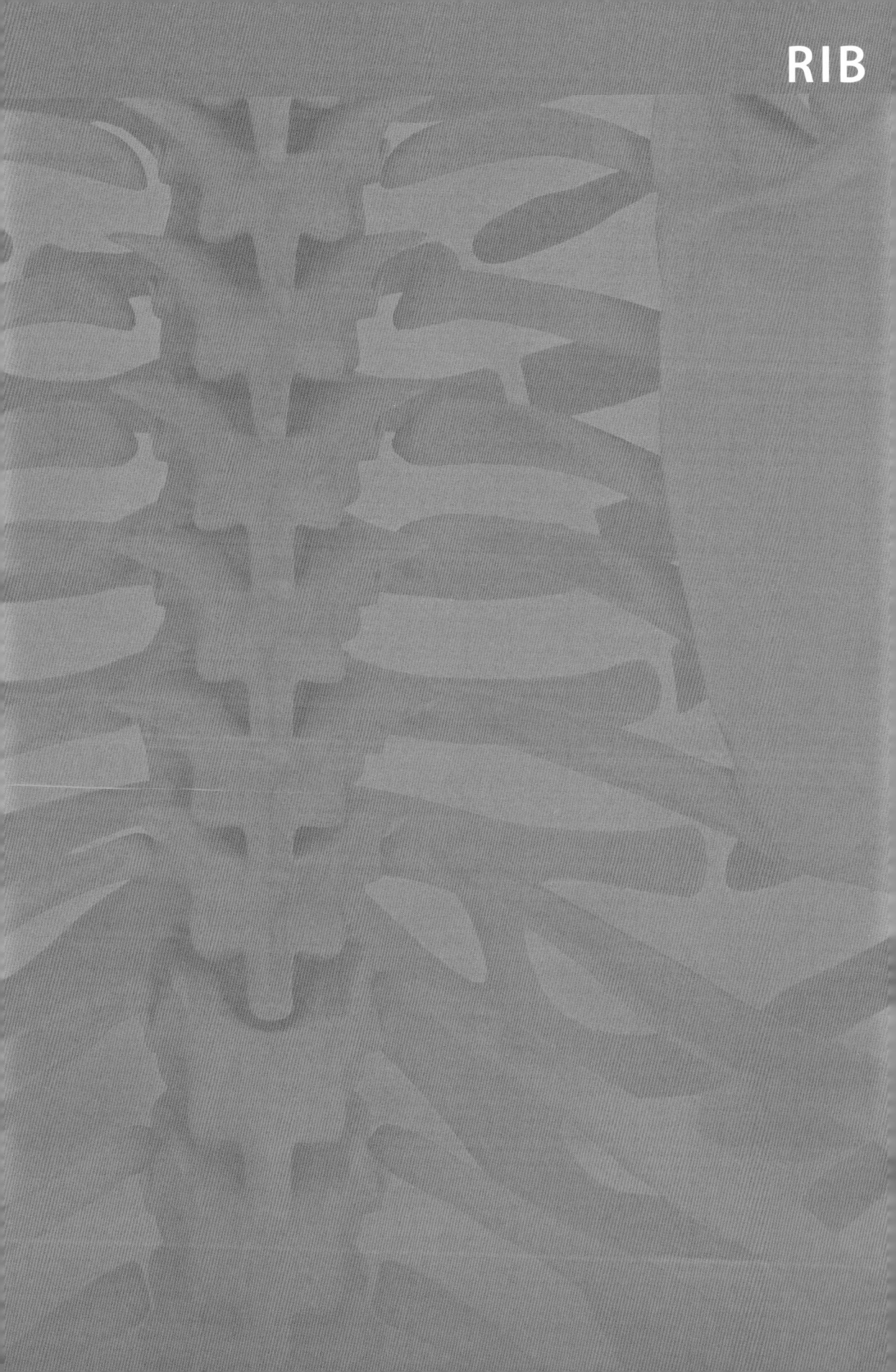

RIB

Diagnosis: Exhaled Rib

Example: Right Rib 5 Exhaled

- ◆ Patient position: Sitting. Extend left arm (contralateral to side of diagnosis) at the shoulder, having the patient hold onto the table to lock out the left side and stabilize the barrier.

- ◆ Index finger monitors the superior aspect of right (ipsilateral to side of diagnosis) rib 5 posteriorly.

- ◆ Middle finger monitors T5 transverse process on left (contralateral to side of diagnosis).

- ◆ Long lever: Right (ipsilateral to side of diagnosis) upper extremity.

- ◆ Engage the barrier: While extending the elbow, flex, adduct, and externally rotate the arm at the shoulder to engage motion specifically at rib 5 and T5. Add an inferior force to rib 5 to encourage motion toward inhalation.

Note: The degree of flexion, adduction, and external rotation will depend on the level of the dysfunctional rib.

- ◆ Treatment is complete when the dysfunctional rib (rib 5) has moved through all pseudo-barriers and the final barrier. This is followed by palpation of the PRM at the level of the dysfunction (rib 5) coordinated with surrounding ribs (ribs 4 and 6) and thoracic vertebrae (T4 and T5).

- ◆ Conclusion: Ease the patient out of the engaged position, providing support back to neutral. Releasing the first 15 degrees back to neutral should be done slowly to avoid retriggering the somatic dysfunction.

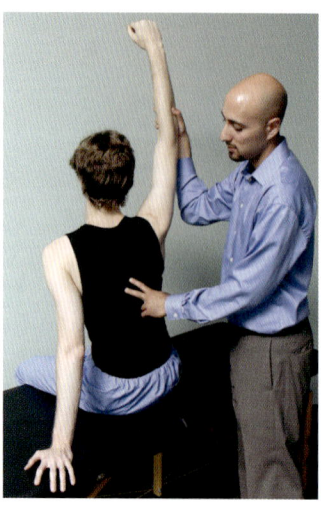 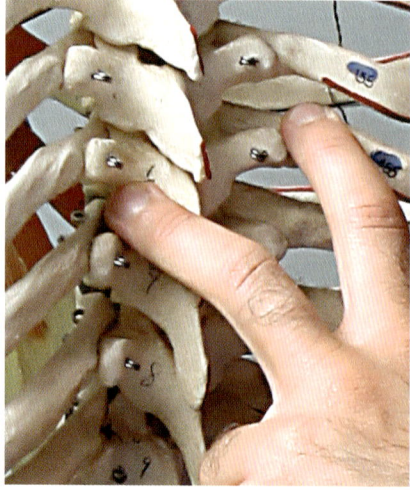

Diagnosis: Inhaled Rib

Example: Right Rib 5 Inhaled

- Patient position: Sitting. Extend left shoulder (contralateral to side of diagnosis), having the patient hold onto the table to lock out the left side and stabilize the barrier.

- Index finger monitors the inferior aspect of rib 5 posteriorly.

- Middle finger monitors the T5 transverse process on the left (contralateral to side of diagnosis).

- Long lever: Right (ipsilateral to side of diagnosis) upper extremity.

- Engage the barrier: While extending the elbow, extend and internally rotate the arm through contact at the wrist to engage motion specifically at rib 5 and T5. Add a superior force to rib 5 to encourage motion toward exhalation.

Note: The degree of extension and internal rotation will depend on the level of the dysfunctional rib.

- Treatment is complete when the dysfunctional rib (rib 5) has moved through all pseudo-barriers and the final barrier. This is followed by palpation of the PRM at the level of the dysfunction (rib 5) coordinated with surrounding ribs (ribs 4 and 6) and vertebrae (T4 and T5).

- Conclusion: Ease the patient out of the engaged position, providing support back to neutral. Releasing the first 15 degrees back to neutral should be done slowly to avoid retriggering the somatic dysfunction.

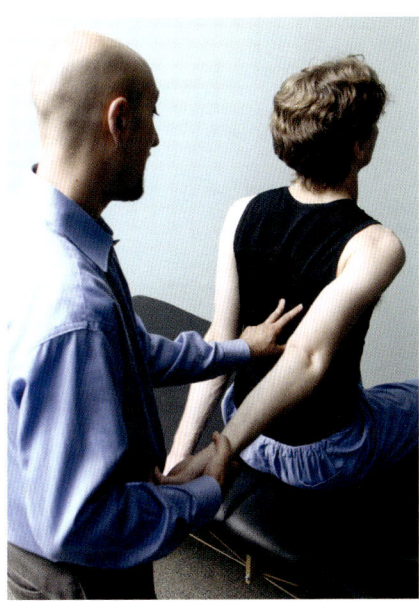
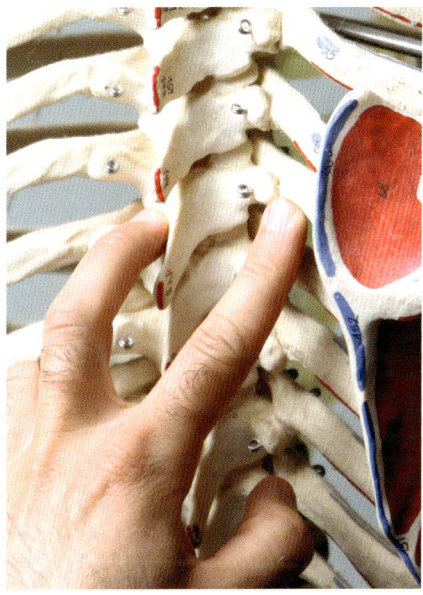

RIB

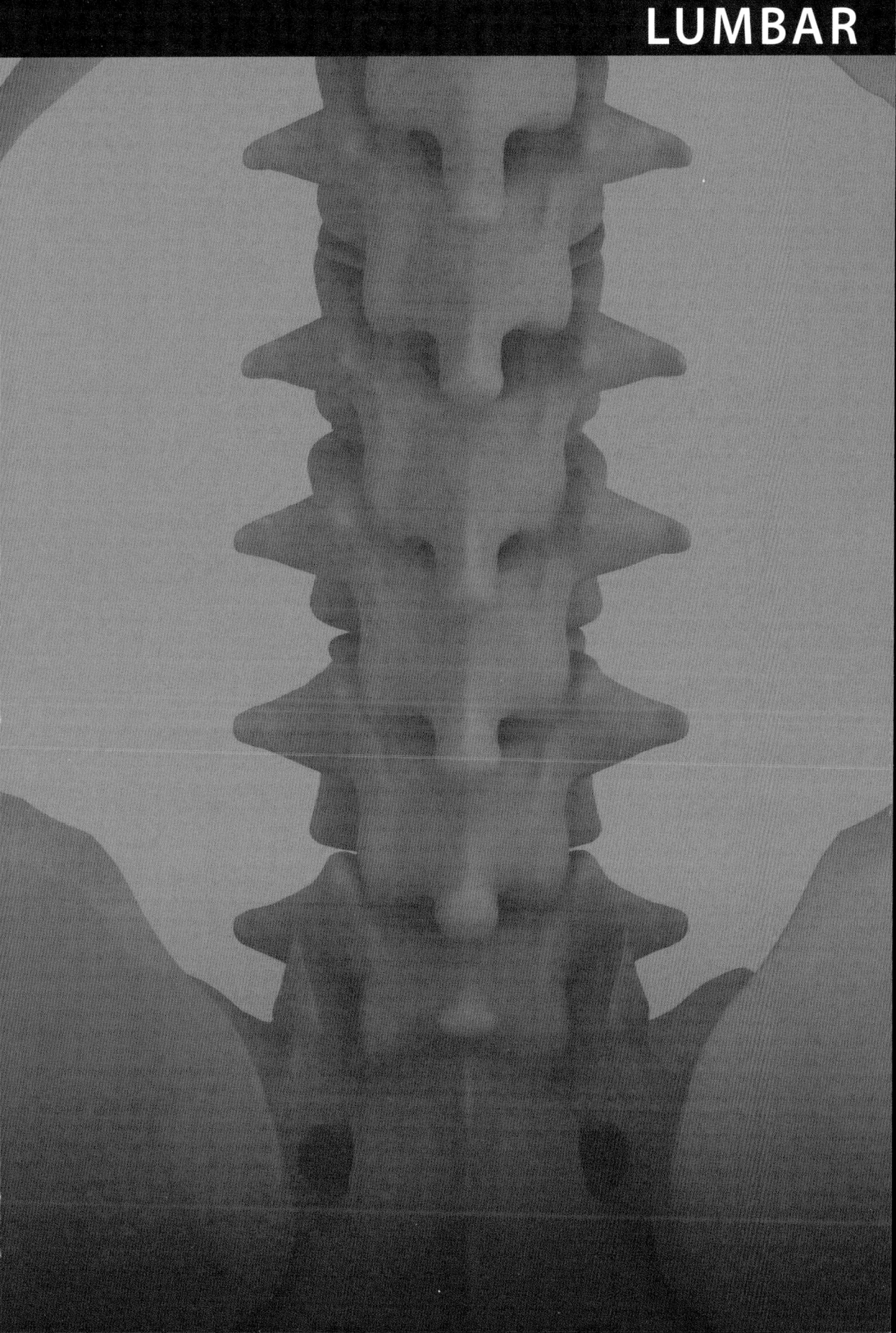

Diagnosis: L4ERS$_L$ (Extended, Rotated and Sidebent Left)

Treatment position: L4FRS$_R$ (Flexed, Rotated and Sidebent Right)

- Patient position: Prone.

- Index finger monitors right transverse or spinous process (contralateral to side of diagnosis) of vertebra above (L3) for entire setup and treatment.

- Engage the barrier: Flex and abduct the right lower extremity (contralateral to side of diagnosis) at the hip with knee bent approximately 90 degrees, localizing motion to the barrier. This induces right rotation of the dysfunctional vertebra (L4) relative to the neutral vertebra (L3). With left knee bent, operator abducts the left hip until motion is localized to engage the dysfunctional vertebra (L4) relative to the above vertebra (L3).

- Long lever: Left lower extremity (ipsilateral to side of diagnosis). Internally rotate the hip by taking the foot laterally and cephalad to lock out the barrier. This uses two planes of motion to localize the barrier more accurately. Maintain appropriate pressure at the right transverse process of the neutral vertebra (L3) to prevent it from rotating right.

- Treatment is complete when the dysfunctional vertebra (L4) has moved through all pseudo-barriers and the final barrier. This is followed by palpation of the PRM at the level of the dysfunction (L4) coordinated with surrounding vertebrae (L3 and L5).

- Conclusion: Ease the patient out of the engaged position, providing support back to neutral. Releasing the first 15 degrees back to neutral should be done slowly to avoid retriggering the somatic dysfunction.

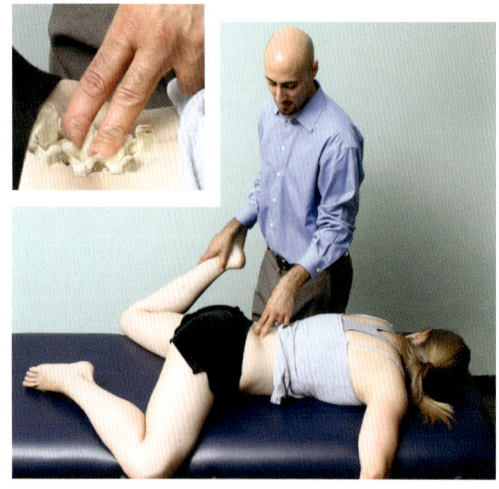
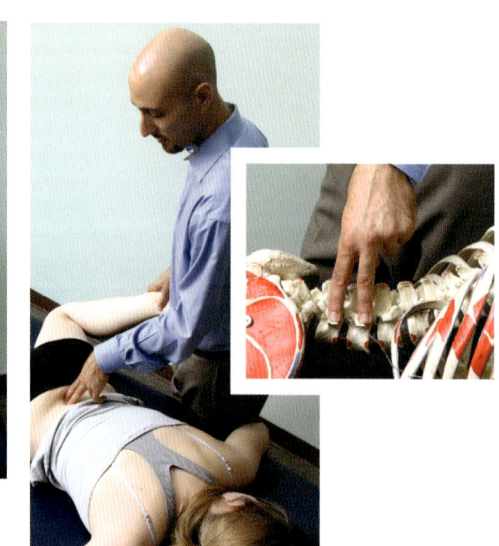

Diagnosis: L4FRS$_L$ (Flexed, Rotated and Sidebent Left)

Treatment position: L4ERS$_R$ (Extended, Rotated and Sidebent Right)

- Patient position: Prone, on elbows to induce extension from above (i.e., prone prop position). Induces right lumbar sidebending (contralateral to side of diagnosis) by drawing both lower extremities laterally to the right.

- Monitor at right (contralateral to side of diagnosis) transverse processes of L3 and L4 for entire setup and treatment. Firmly stabilize right transverse or spinous process of the above vertebra (L3) in place, preventing right rotation.

- Long lever: Extended right lower extremity (contralateral to side of diagnosis).

- Engage the barrier: Support right lower extremity (contralateral to side of diagnosis) proximal to the knee. Introduce extension at the hip until motion is localized at the dysfunctional vertebra (L4). Adduct and externally rotate the right lower extremity to engage right rotation of the dysfunctional vertebra (L4).

- Treatment is complete when the dysfunctional vertebra (L4) has moved through all pseudo-barriers and the final barrier. This is followed by palpation of the PRM at the level of the dysfunction (L4) coordinated with surrounding vertebrae (L3 and L5).

- Conclusion: Ease the patient out of the engaged position, providing support back to neutral. Releasing the first 15 degrees back to neutral should be done slowly to avoid retriggering the somatic dysfunction.

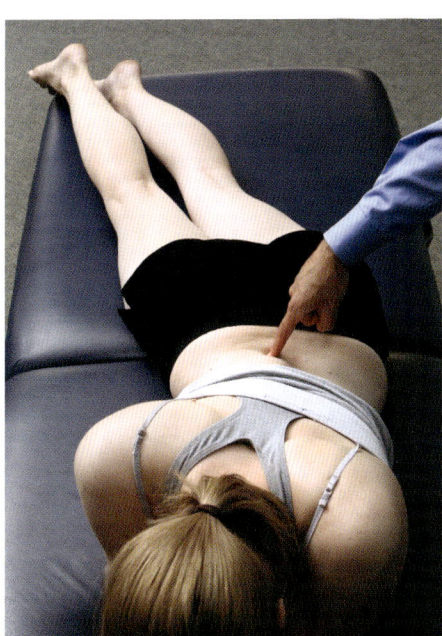 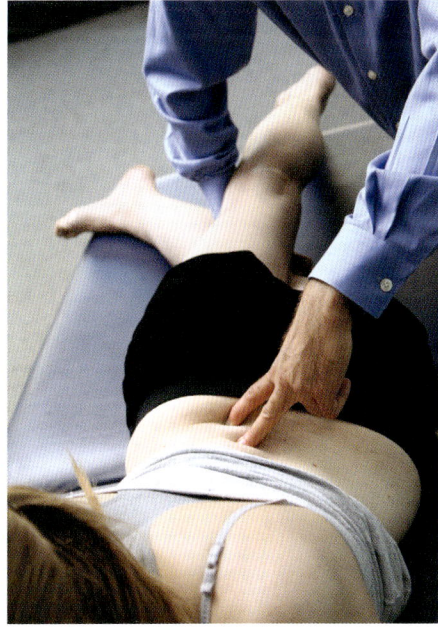

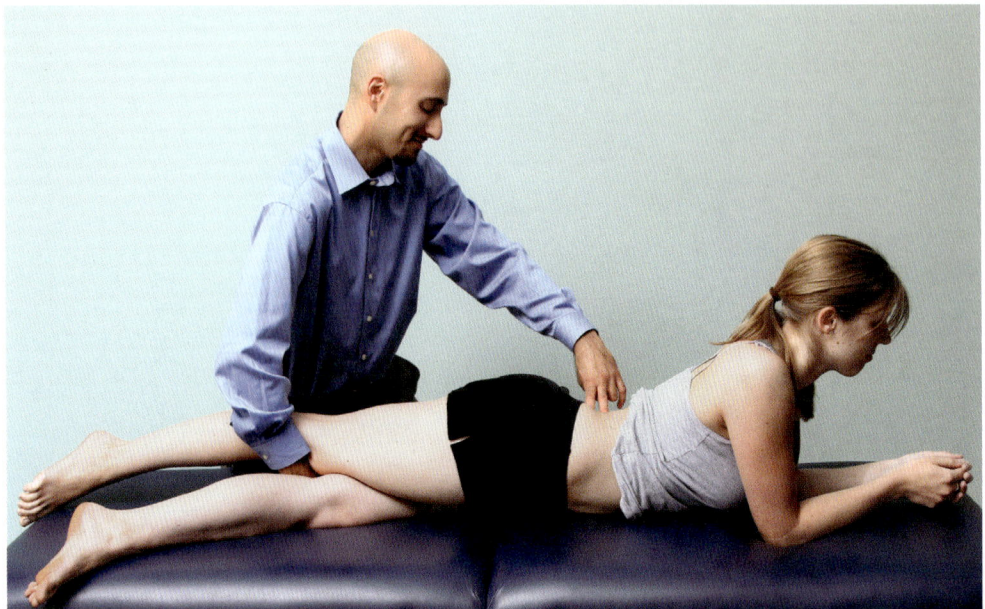

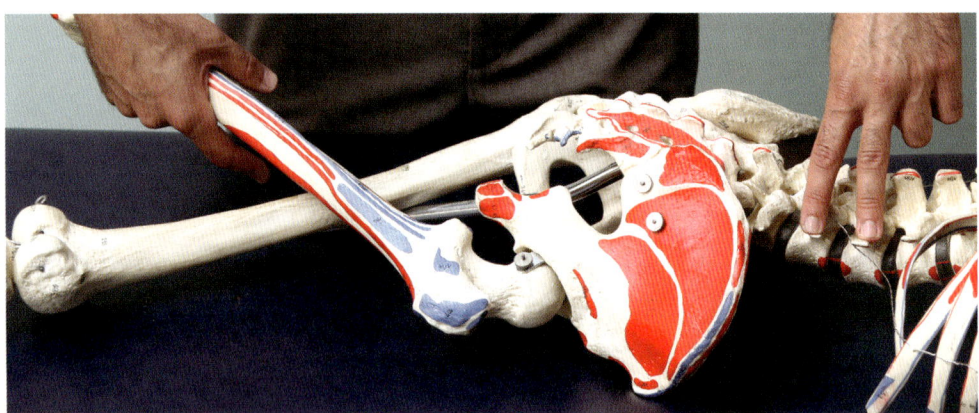

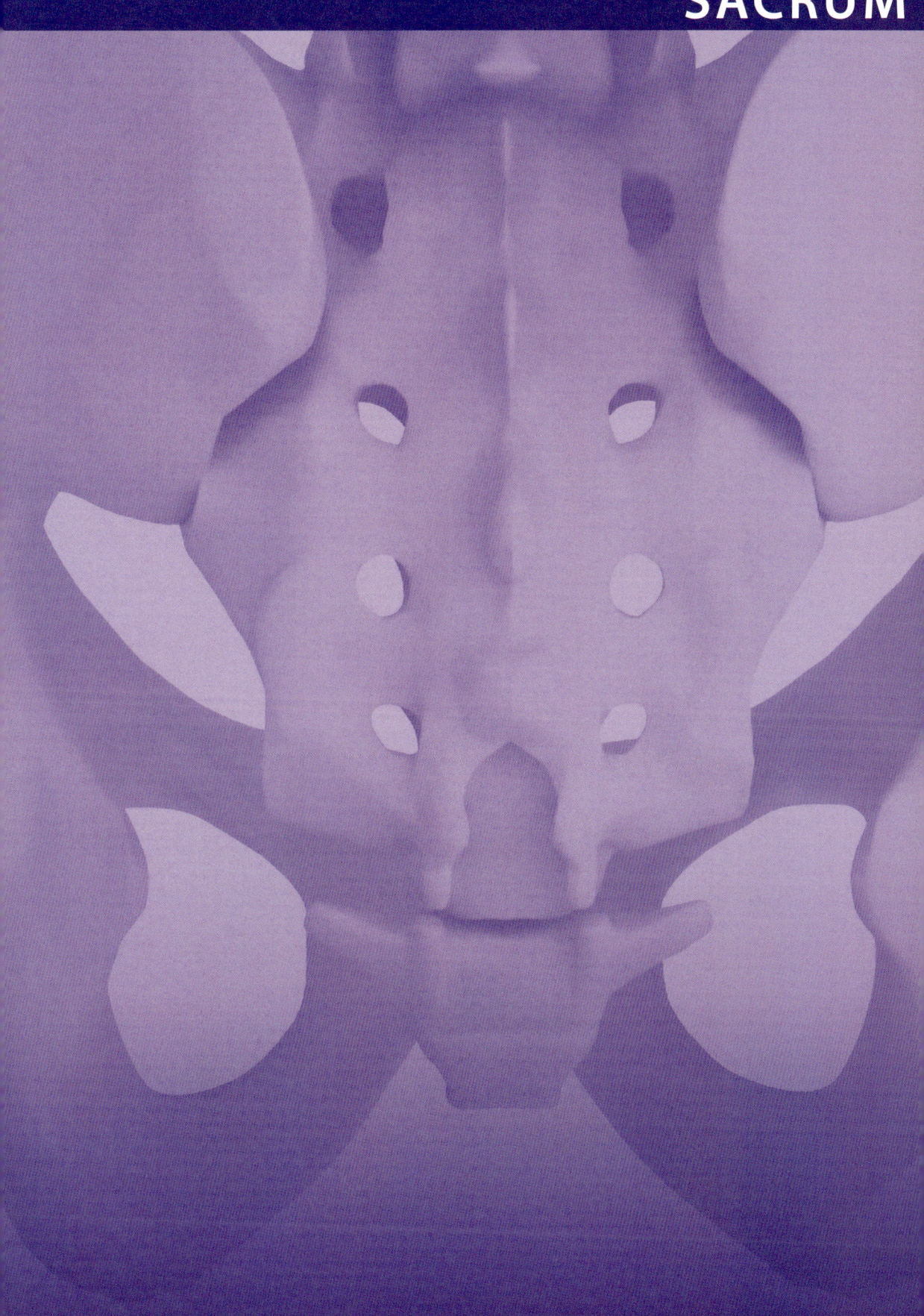

Diagnosis: Forward Torsion

Sacral Rotation Ipsilateral to Oblique Axis

Example: Left on Left Sacral Torsion

- Patient position: Prone with arms hanging off the sides of the table (i.e., modified Sims' position). Operator stands to the patient's right (contralateral to side of axis).

- Engage the barrier: Flex the knees and hips. Rotate sacrum to the right with axis side down. Monitor for flexion and extension at the lumbosacral junction. Using a three-finger approach, monitor with one finger on the right sacral base, one finger on the right transverse or spinous process of L5, and one finger stabilizing the right ilium to encourage the anterior right sacral base to move posteriorly.

- Long lever: Both lower extremities. Apply pressure at the patient's legs distal to the knees directed toward the floor to induce sacral rotation. Make sure not to induce rotation of L5 while adjusting the long lever.

- Treatment is complete when the right sacral base moves posteriorly through all pseudo-barriers and the final barrier. This is followed by palpation of the PRM at the sacrum coordinated with the pelvis and lumbar vertebrae.

- Conclusion: Ease the patient out of the engaged position, providing support back to neutral. Releasing the first 15 degrees back to neutral should be done slowly to avoid retriggering the somatic dysfunction.

Note: Patient may require a pillow under lower thigh or knee for comfort.

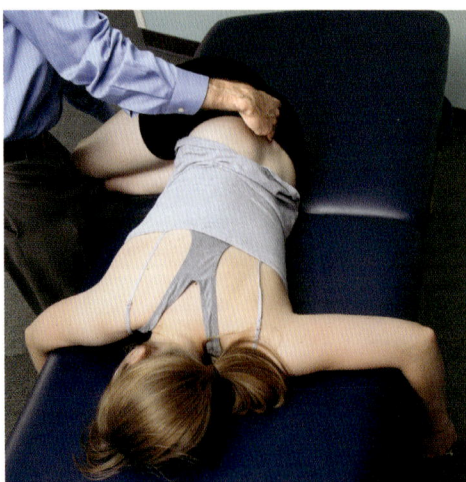
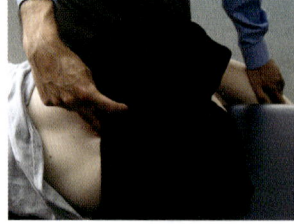
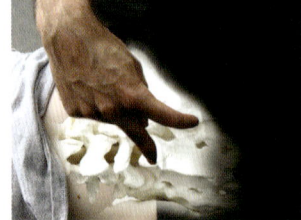

Diagnosis: Backward Torsion

Sacral Rotation Contralateral to Oblique Axis

Example: Left on Right Sacral Torsion

- Patient position: Right lateral recumbent (ipsilateral to side of axis, i.e., axis side down).

- Engage the barrier: Extend the lower extremities below the dysfunction, and extend the spine above the dysfunction. Patient extends arm and grasps the table for stabilization. Operator sits anterior to the patient's right knee, maintaining extension of the right lower extremity. Monitor with index finger on left sacral base and middle finger on L5 left transverse or spinous process. Firmly stabilize L5 spinous process from rotating, to encourage the posterior left sacral base to move anteriorly.

- Long lever: Left lower extremity. Flex and adduct the patient's left hip and knee to more specifically engage the sacrum and pelvis.

- Treatment is complete when the left sacral base has moved anteriorly through all pseudo-barriers and the final barrier. This is followed by palpation of the PRM at the sacrum coordinated with the pelvis and lumbar vertebrae.

- Conclusion: Ease the patient out of the engaged position, providing support back to neutral. Releasing the first 15 degrees back to neutral should be done slowly to avoid retriggering the somatic dysfunction.

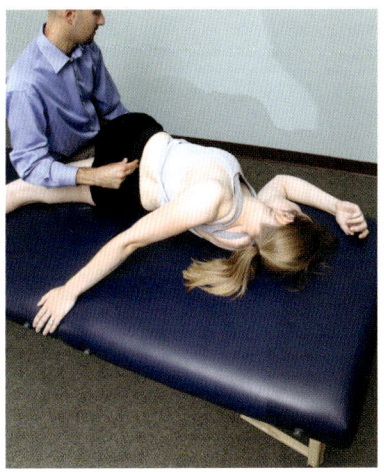 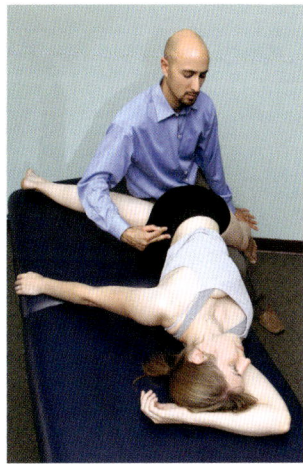 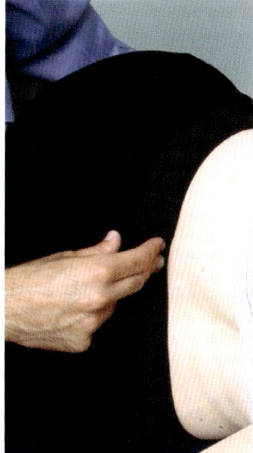

Diagnosis: Unilateral Extension

Example: Right Sacral Extension

- Patient position: Prone.

- Engage the barrier: With the heel of one hand monitoring and stabilizing the right (ipsilateral to side of diagnosis) sacral base, apply pressure anteriorly. With the other hand, hold the patient's right foot, flex at the knee, internally rotate the lower extremity, and abduct the hip to gap the sacroiliac joint. Proper hand positioning at the foot and flexion of the knee stabilize the ankle, knee, and hip.

- Long levers: (1) Right lower extremity (ipsilateral to side of diagnosis). (2) Force created by the operator's hand applying anterior pressure to the posterior sacral base.

- Treatment is complete when the right sacral base has moved anteriorly through all pseudo-barriers and the final barrier. This is followed by palpation of the PRM at the sacrum coordinated with the pelvis.

- Conclusion: Ease the patient out of the engaged position, providing support back to neutral. Releasing the first 15 degrees back to neutral should be done slowly to avoid retriggering the somatic dysfunction.

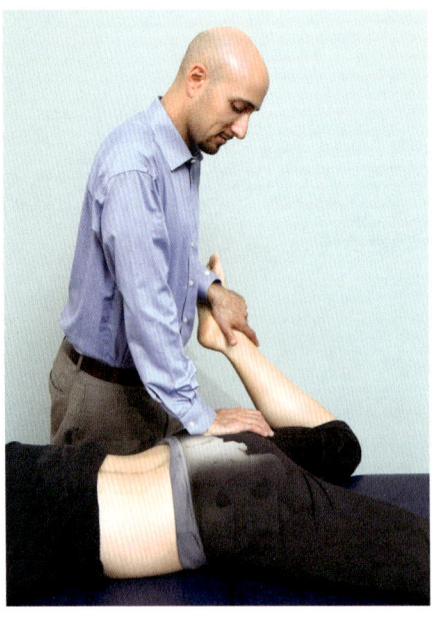 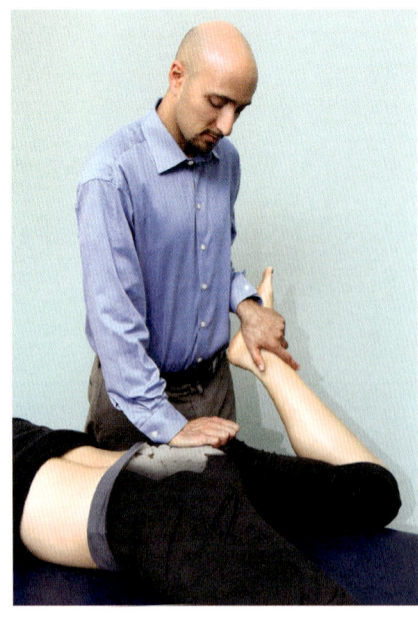

SACRUM

Diagnosis: Unilateral Flexion

Example: Left Sacral Flexion

- Patient position: Prone.

- Engage the barrier: With the heel of one hand monitoring and stabilizing the left (ipsilateral to side of diagnosis) posterior ILA (inferior lateral angle), apply pressure anteriorly. With the other hand, hold the patient's left foot, flex the knee, and internally rotate and abduct the hip to localize to the area of greatest restriction between the sacrum and ilium. Proper hand positioning at the foot and flexion of the knee stabilize the ankle, knee, and hip.

- Long levers: (1) Left lower extremity (ipsilateral to side of diagnosis). (2) Force created by the operator's hand applying anterior pressure to the posterior ILA.

- Treatment is complete when the left ILA has moved anteriorly through all pseudo-barriers and the final barrier. This is followed by palpation of the PRM at the sacrum coordinated with the pelvis.

- Conclusion: Ease the patient out of the engaged position, providing support back to neutral. Releasing the first 15 degrees back to neutral should be done slowly to avoid retriggering the somatic dysfunction.

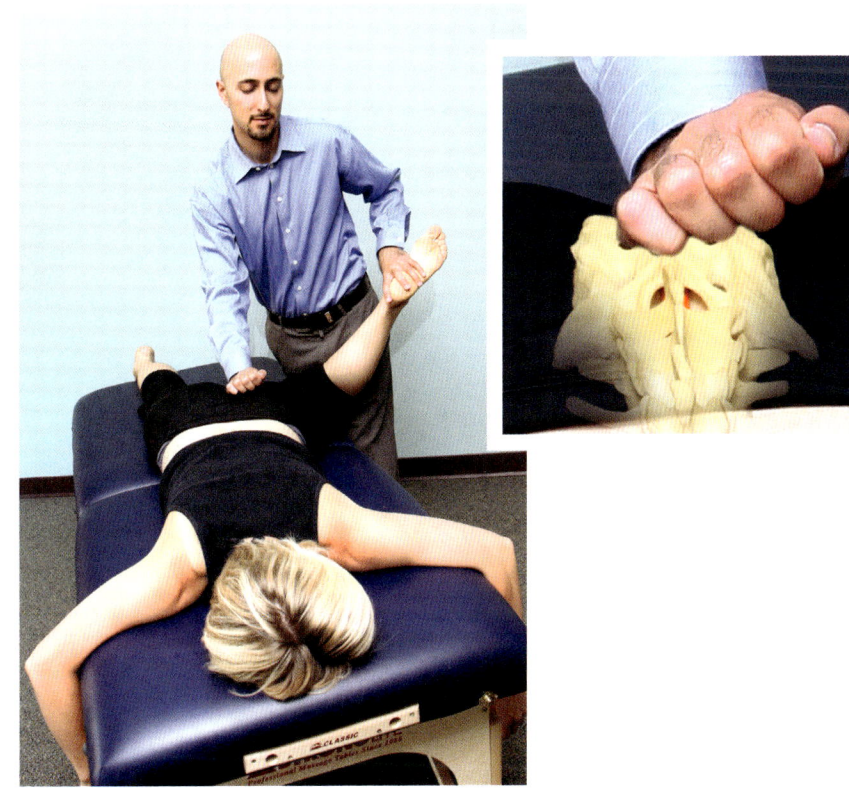

Diagnosis: Bilateral Extension

Example: Bilateral Sacral Extension

- ◆ Patient position: Prone, knees together, propped on elbows (sphinx position).

- ◆ Engage the barrier: With the heel of one hand monitoring and stabilizing the bilateral posterior sacral base, apply pressure anteriorly. With the other hand, hold the patient's feet and introduce flexion through the knees. This creates anterior rotation of bilateral innominates to stabilize the innominates. Proper hand positioning at the feet and flexion of the knees stabilize the ankles, knees, and hips. Patient assists with exhalation.

- ◆ Long levers: (1) Through the bilaterally flexed knees with operator holding the feet. (2) Force created by the operator's hand applying anterior pressure to the bilateral posterior sacral base.

- ◆ Treatment is complete when the bilateral posterior sacral base has moved anteriorly through all pseudo-barriers and the final barrier. This is followed by palpation of the PRM at the sacrum, coordinated with the pelvis and lumbars.

- ◆ Conclusion: Ease the patient out of the engaged position, providing support back to neutral. Releasing the first 15 degrees back to neutral should be done slowly to avoid retriggering the somatic dysfunction.

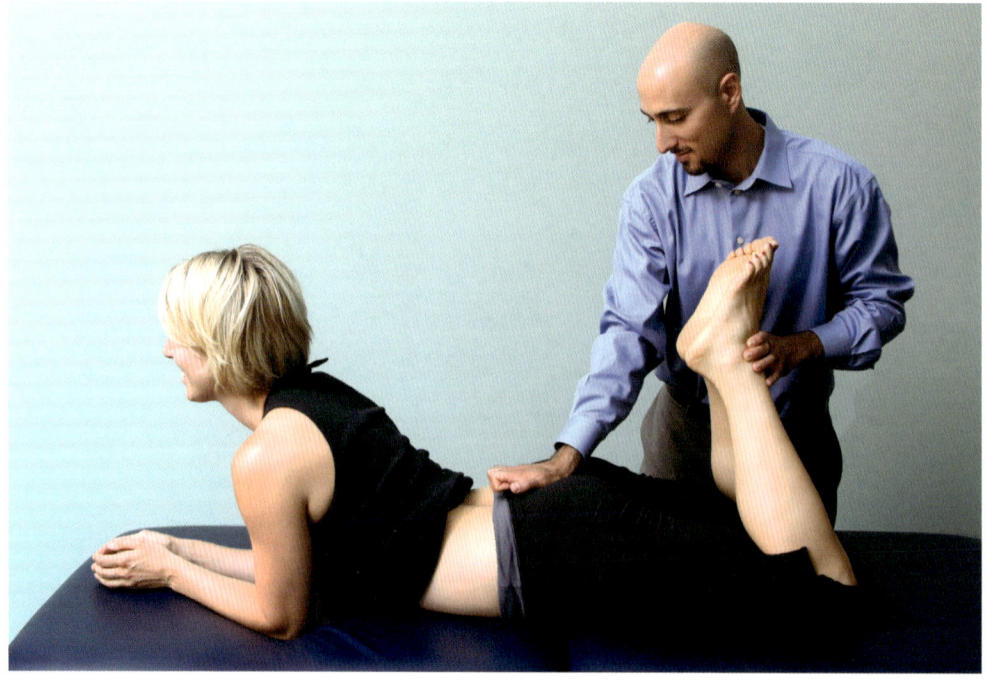

SACRUM

Diagnosis: Bilateral Flexion

Example: Bilateral Sacral Flexion

- ◆ Patient position: Seated on table with legs extended directly in front.

- ◆ Operator applies anterior pressure to the sacral apex, encouraging sacral extension with finger pads. Heel of hand will monitor lumbars.

- ◆ Engage the barrier: With the heel of one hand monitoring the lumbar spine, the finger pads apply anterior pressure to the sacral apex, encouraging sacral extension. Use the heel of this hand to monitor for lumbar flexion applied by the other hand from above. With this hand, introduce flexion of the spine with careful engagement of the barrier using the patient's cervicodorsal area.

- ◆ Long levers: (1) Flexion through the spine and patient's cervicodorsal area. Be gentle with the amount of pressure and flexion introduced through the patient's head. The dura is vulnerable to aggressive and/or too much flexion. (2) Force created by the operator's hand applying anterior pressure to the bilaterally posterior sacral apex.

- ◆ Treatment is complete when the posterior sacral apex has moved anteriorly through all pseudo-barriers and the final barrier. This is followed by palpation of the PRM at the sacrum, coordinated with the pelvis and lumbars.

- ◆ Conclusion: Ease the patient out of the engaged position, providing support back to neutral. Releasing the first 15 degrees back to neutral should be done slowly to avoid retriggering the somatic dysfunction.

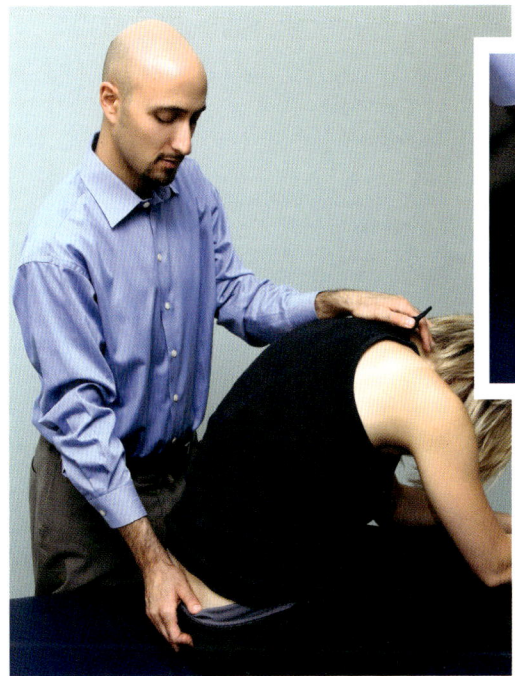
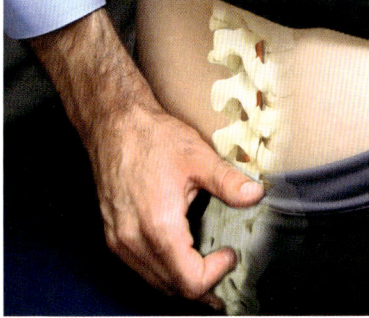

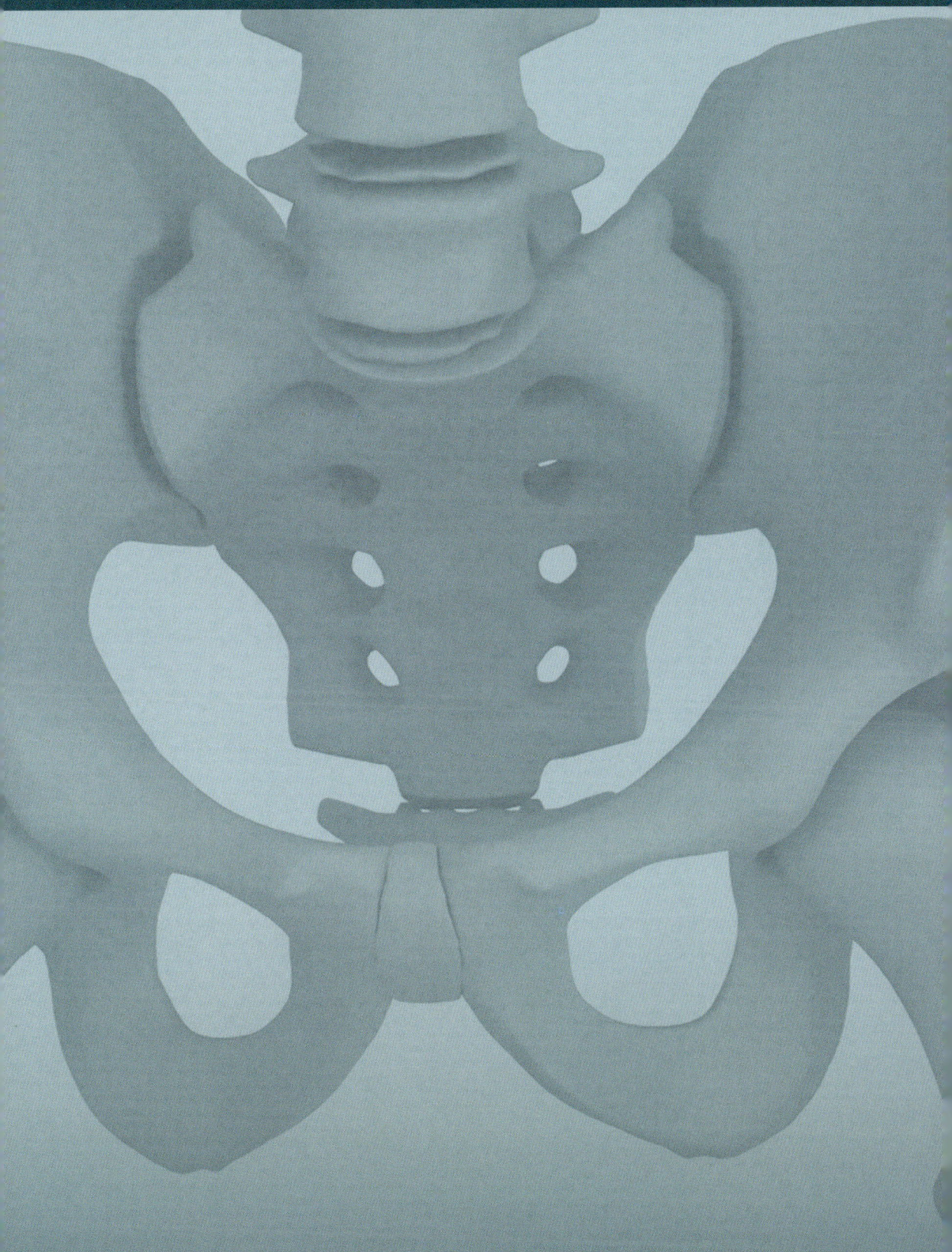

Diagnosis: Superior Innominate Shear (Upslip)

Example: Left Superior Innominate Shear

- ◆ Patient position: Prone.

- ◆ Throughout the procedure, maintain awareness of motion at posterior sacroiliac joint.

- ◆ Engage the barrier: Holding the patient's left foot (ipsilateral to side of diagnosis), internally rotate and abduct the left hip to gap the posterior aspect of the sacroiliac joint. Proper hand positioning at the foot and flexion of the knee stabilize the ankle, knee, and hip.

- ◆ Long lever: Left lower extremity (ipsilateral to side of diagnosis). Maintain traction of the lower extremity for release of the posterior sacroiliac joint. The patient assists with slow, deep breathing.

- ◆ Treatment is complete when the dysfunctional (left) innominate moves inferiorly through all pseudo-barriers and the final barrier. This is followed by palpation of the PRM through the pelvis, left lower extremity, and sacrum.

- ◆ Conclusion: Ease the patient out of the engaged position, providing support back to neutral. Releasing the first 15 degrees back to neutral should be done slowly to avoid retriggering the somatic dysfunction.

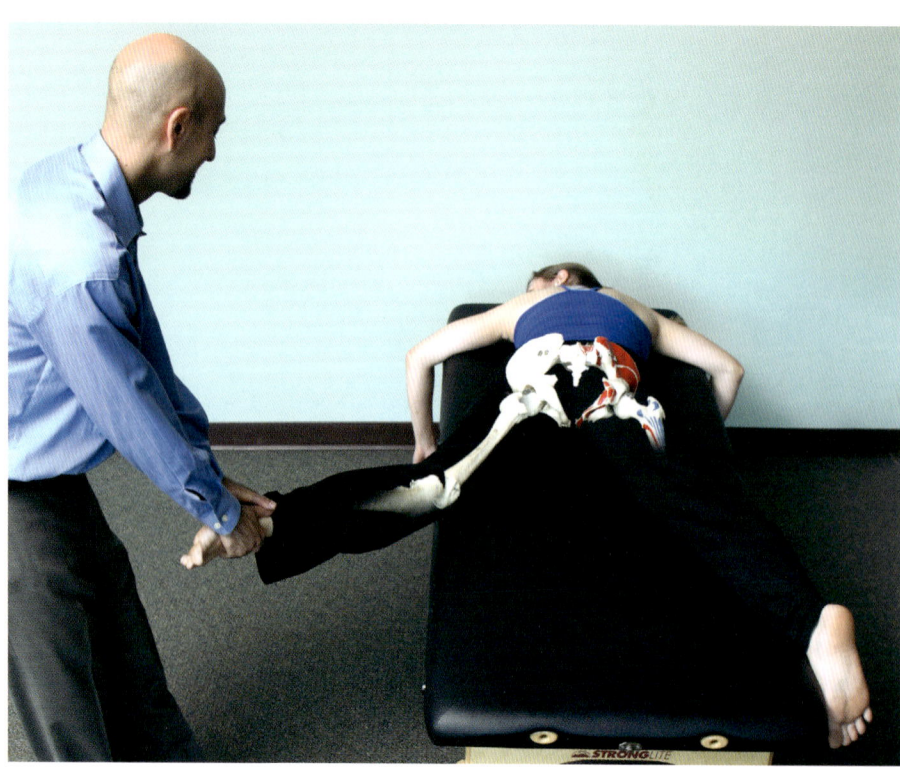

PELVIS

Diagnosis: Inferior Innominate Shear (Downslip)

Example: Left Inferior Innominate Shear

- Patient position: Prone. Dorsum of right foot (contralateral to side of diagnosis) pressing on the end of the table. Right hand holding the top of the table.

- Engage the barrier: Patient simultaneously pulls inferiorly with the right hand (contralateral to side of diagnosis) and dorsiflexes the right foot against the treatment table. This combination stabilizes the right innominate and sacrum. Monitor at left ischium (ipsilateral to side of diagnosis). Flex the left knee and internally rotate the left hip to gap the sacroiliac joint. Encourage superior motion of the innominate with ischial contact.

- Long levers: (1) Left lower extremity (ipsilateral to side of diagnosis). (2) Force created by the operator's hand applying superior pressure to the inferior left ischium.

- Treatment is complete when the dysfunctional (left) innominate moves superiorly through all pseudo-barriers and the final barrier. This is followed by palpation of the PRM through the pelvis, left lower extremity, and sacrum.

- Conclusion: Ease the patient out of the engaged position, providing support back to neutral. Releasing the first 15 degrees back to neutral should be done slowly to avoid retriggering the somatic dysfunction.

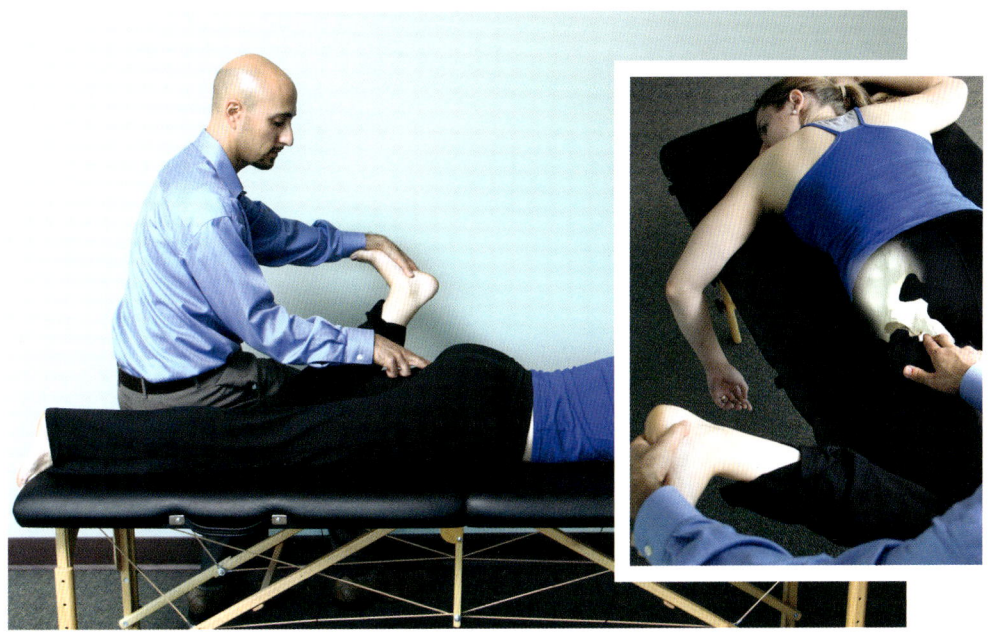

Diagnosis: Anterior Innominate Rotation

Example: Left Anterior Innominate Rotation

- Patient position: Supine.

- Throughout the procedure, maintain awareness of motion at pubic symphysis and SI joint.

- Engage the barrier: Adduct the right lower extremity (contralateral to side of diagnosis). Flex the left knee and hip (ipsilateral to side of diagnosis), taking the lower extremity to the right shoulder. This assists in gapping the pubic symphysis and/or the SI joint. Externally rotate the tibia from the left heel.

- Long lever: Left lower extremity (ipsilateral to side of diagnosis). Proper hand positioning at the heel and forearm contact at the knee stabilize the ankle, knee, and hip.

- Treatment is complete when the dysfunctional (left) innominate moves posteriorly through all pseudo-barriers and the final barrier. This is followed by palpation of the PRM through the left lower extremity, pubic symphysis, and SI joint, coordinated with the surrounding structures.

- Conclusion: Ease the patient out of the engaged position, providing support back to neutral. Releasing the first 15 degrees back to neutral should be done slowly to avoid retriggering the somatic dysfunction.

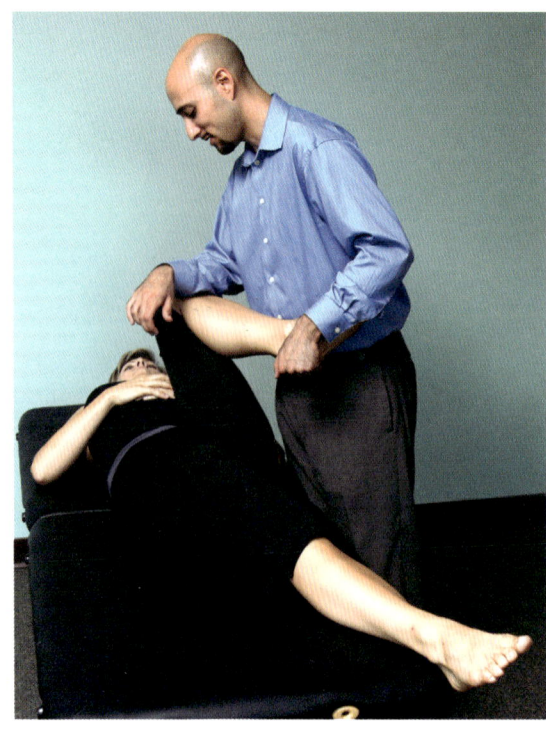

Diagnosis: Posterior Innominate Rotation

Example: Left Posterior Innominate Rotation

- Patient position: Supine.

- Monitor for motion at the left anterior superior iliac spine (ASIS) (ipsilateral to side of diagnosis) and across the pubic symphysis.

- Engage the barrier: Stabilize the right lower extremity (contralateral to side of diagnosis) by abducting the right hip, flexing the knee, and allowing the lateral aspect of the foot to rest on the table. Extend the left knee (ipsilateral to side of diagnosis), abduct the leg, and externally rotate at the hip from the foot.

- Long lever: Left lower extremity (ipsilateral to side of diagnosis). Proper hand positioning at the foot stabilizes the ankle, knee, and hip.

- Treatment is complete when the dysfunctional (left) innominate moves anteriorly through all pseudo-barriers and the final barrier. This is followed by palpation of the PRM through the left lower extremity, pubic symphysis, and SI joint, coordinated with the surrounding structures.

- Conclusion: Ease the patient out of the engaged position, providing support back to neutral. Releasing the first 15 degrees back to neutral should be done slowly to avoid retriggering the somatic dysfunction.

Note: If having difficulty locking out the right lower extremity (contralateral to side of diagnosis), consider inducing further external rotation by weighing down the right knee or adding a pillow under the right foot.

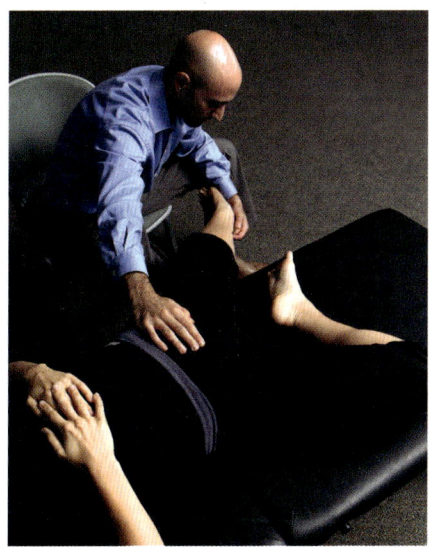

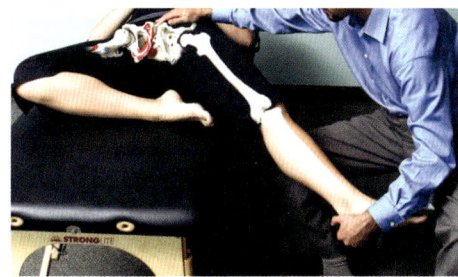

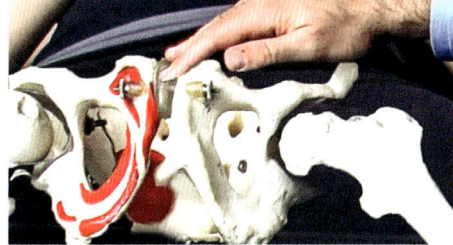

Diagnosis: Inflare

Example: Left Inflare

- ◆ Patient position: Supine.

- ◆ Right thumb monitors for motion at the right pubis (contralateral to side of diagnosis). Stabilize the right ASIS with right hand.

- ◆ Engage the barrier: Holding the left heel (ipsilateral to side of diagnosis), abduct the hip while flexing the hip and knee. Operator's abdomen is used as a fulcrum against the knee. Proper hand positioning at the heel stabilizes the ankle, knee, and hip.

- ◆ Long lever: Left lower extremity (ipsilateral to side of diagnosis).

- ◆ Treatment is complete when the dysfunctional (left) innominate moves through all pseudo-barriers and the final barrier. This is followed by palpation of the PRM at the pubis, coordinated with the surrounding structures.

- ◆ Conclusion: Ease the patient out of the engaged position, providing support back to neutral. Releasing the first 15 degrees back to neutral should be done slowly to avoid retriggering the somatic dysfunction.

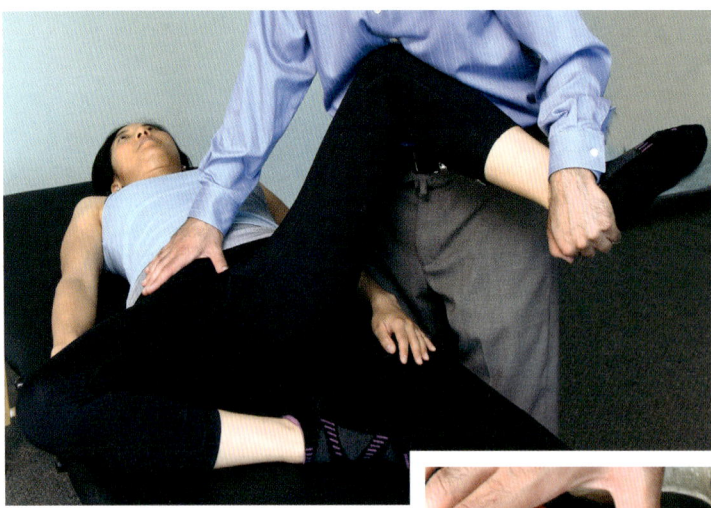

Diagnosis: Outflare

Example: Left Outflare

- Patient position: Supine.

- Right thumb monitors the right pubis (contralateral to side of diagnosis). Stabilize the right ASIS with right hand.

- Engage the barrier: Holding the left heel (ipsilateral to side of diagnosis), flex, adduct, and internally rotate the hip. Flex the knee from the heel using the operator's shoulder as a fulcrum against the knee. Proper hand positioning at the heel stabilizes the ankle, knee, and hip.

- Long lever: Left lower extremity (ipsilateral to side of diagnosis).

- Treatment is complete when the dysfunctional (left) innominate moves through all pseudo-barriers and the final barrier. This is followed by palpation of the PRM at the pubis, coordinated with the surrounding structures.

- Conclusion: Ease the patient out of the engaged position, providing support back to neutral. Releasing the first 15 degrees back to neutral should be done slowly to avoid retriggering the somatic dysfunction.

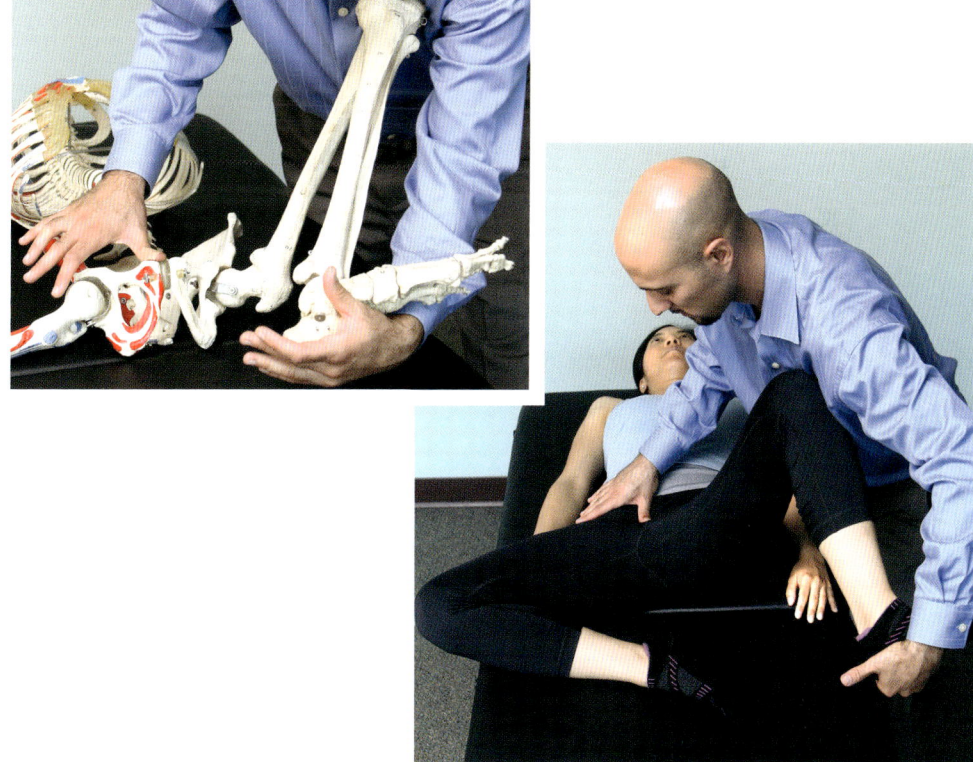

PART 3

Coccyx and Craniococcygeal Anatomy

BOBBY NOURANI, DO, FAAO

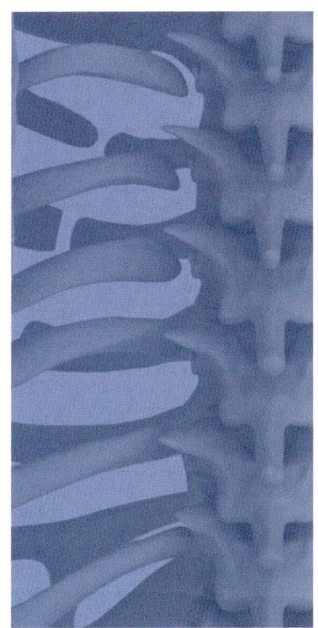
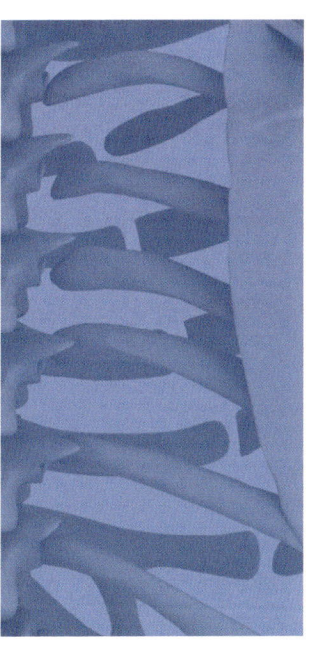
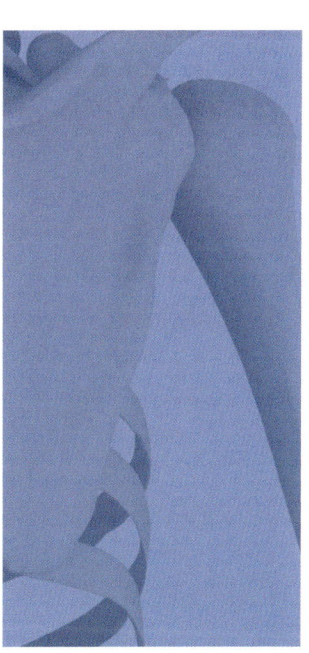

Treatment of Coccydynia with the Long Lever Technique, and Craniococcygeal Interrelated Anatomy

The principles of Long Lever Technique can be applied to different anatomical regions and bones, including the bony coccyx and coccygeal region. The following sections review coccydynia evaluation and treatment, associated anatomy, and craniococcygeal continuity and interrelationships.

Coccydynia

Coccydynia (or coccygodynia, coccyalgia) is a debilitating pain of the coccygeal region that substantially impacts quality of life. It is common in primary and musculoskeletal care and can be challenging to treat (Lirette et al. 2014). The etiology is multifactorial; the most common cause is trauma, including falls and childbirth (Lirette et al. 2014; Schapiro 1950), but also prolonged direct sacral pressure sitting on hard surfaces (Pennekamp et al. 2005). Nontraumatic causes also contribute (Kerr, Benson, and Schrot 2011; Lirette et al. 2014; Nathan, Fisher, and Roberts 2010; Patel, Appannagari, and Whang 2008). Pain may radiate to the pelvic floor, limiting activities of daily living. Dyspareunia and pain with defecation are possible (Lirette et al. 2014; Pennekamp et al. 2005; Schapiro 1950).

Conservative management of coccydynia is successful in 90 percent of patients; treatments include coccygeal cushions, donut cushions, postural training, and nonsteroidal anti-inflammatory drugs (Capar et al. 2007; Thiele 1963; Trollegaard, Aarby, and Hellberg 2010). Treatment options are limited for the refractory 10 percent. A systematic review compared commonly used nonsurgical interventions but did not conclude in favor of any specific intervention (Howard et al. 2013). Coccygectomy is the treatment of last resort; however, treatment success varies and the complication rate is approximately 11 percent (Lirette et al. 2014). Transrectal manual therapeutic options are rarely discussed in the literature but may provide long-term relief (Nourani, Gilbert, and Rabago 2020).

See Table 3.1 for a list of differential diagnoses. A diagnosis of chordoma should not be missed. A chordoma is a primary bone tumor that may occur at the skull base or cervical, thoracic, lumbar, or sacrococcygeal spine. It is a slow-growing sarcoma. Metastasis is relatively common, illustrating the potential importance of early diagnosis. As such, it is important to inquire about the constitutional symptoms that often coincide with malignancy, like weight loss, night sweats, and fatigue. X-ray, CT, and MRI imaging are helpful.

Table 3.1 Differential Diagnoses

SACROCOCCYGEAL DISORDERS	OTHER SPINAL DISORDERS	VISCERAL DISORDERS
Coccygeal Fracture	Chordoma	Endometriosis
Coccygeal Spur	Lumbar Degenerative Disc Disease	Fibroid Uterus
Intracoccygeal Dislocation	Lumbar Facet Arthropathy	Hemorrhoids
Ganglion Impar Dysfunction	Lumbar Spondylolisthesis	Intrapelvic Infection/ Inflammation
Sacral Insufficiency Fracture	Mechanical Low Back Pain	Intrapelvic Malignancy
Sacrococcygeal Dislocation	Spondyloarthropathy	Ovarian Cyst
Sacroiliac Joint Pain	Tethered Cord	Pilonidal Cyst

Anatomy

The following is a review of the relevant craniococcygeal soft tissue and bony anatomy. This section is intended to provide the reader with a brief review of the anatomy, craniococcygeal continuity, and anatomical interrelationships. Anatomical understanding and palpation improve diagnostic evaluation.

1. Coccyx: Consists of three to five bones that are usually fused. The first coccygeal vertebra has two cornua projecting upward that articulate with sacral cornua. The first coccygeal vertebra also has transverse processes that may articulate or fuse with the inferolateral sacral angle completing the fifth sacral foramen containing the fifth sacral spinal nerves on each side. The coccygeal vertebrae Co2–Co5 progressively decrease in size and are usually fused nodules. Their pelvic surfaces are directed upward and forward. In the young, intercoccygeal joints contain thin discs of fibrocartilage between the segments. Coccygeal segments fuse slowly. The first and second coccygeal vertebrae often do not unite until the age of thirty, and the remaining coccygeal segments often ossify in the late teens or twenties.

2. Sacrococcygeal joint: Is a symphysis between the sacral apex and coccygeal base, united by a thin fibrocartilaginous disc that is somewhat thicker in front and behind than laterally. It is supported by anterior, posterior, and lateral sacrococcygeal ligaments. The sacrococcygeal junction fuses in later decades, generally later for females than males. This variation supports the mechanics of labor and ideal sacrococcygeal range of motion as the infant's head engages the pelvic inlet and passes through the pelvic outlet.

3. Lateral sacrococcygeal ligament: Connects the inferolateral sacral angle to the transverse process of the first coccygeal vertebra on each side.

4. Intercornual ligament: Connects the coccygeal cornua with the sacrum on each side.

5. Sacrospinous ligament: Has attachments to the ischial spine and lateral margins of the sacrum and coccyx.

6. Sacrotuberous ligament: Attachments include the posterior superior iliac spine, posterior sacroiliac ligaments, medial aspect of the ischial tuberosity, and lateral margins of the sacrum and coccyx.

Figures 3.1–3.3. Craniococcygeal anatomy. (1) Full diagram. (2) Superior portion. (3) Inferior portion. The red markings in (2) and (3) identify stronger attachment sites.

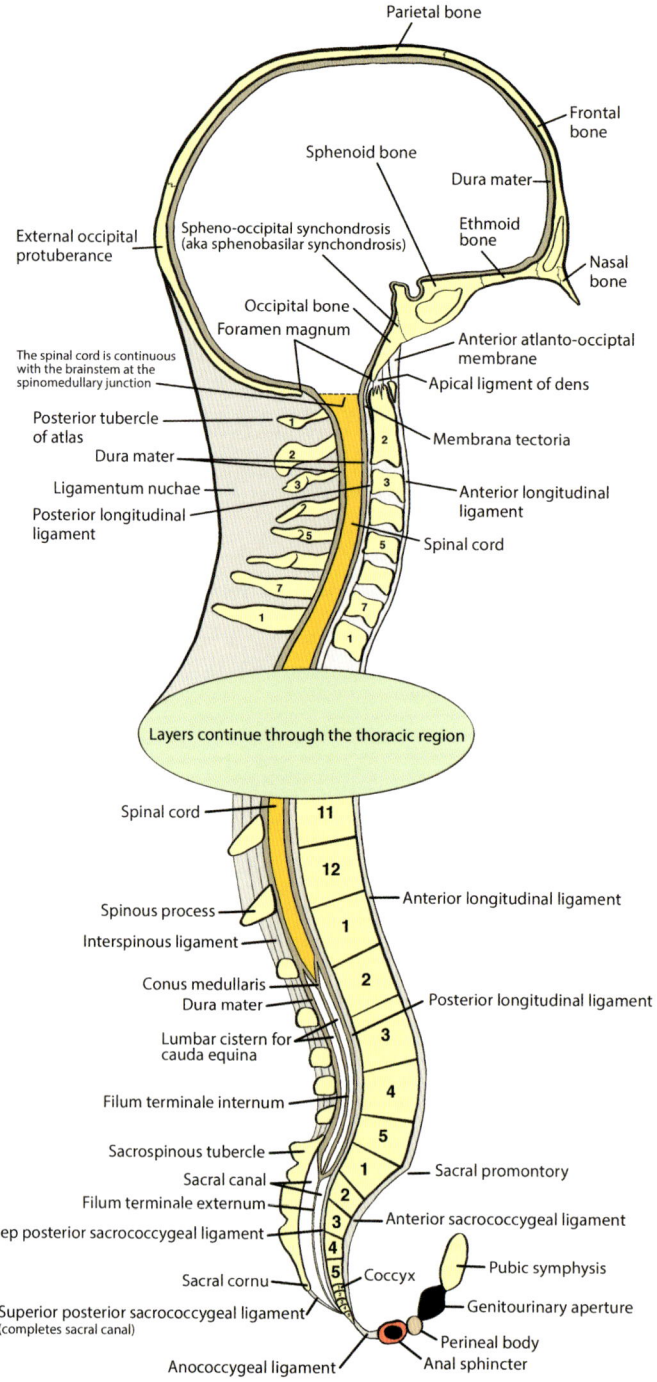

Parietal bone

Frontal bone

Sphenoid bone

Dura mater

External occipital protuberance

Spheno-occipital synchondrosis (aka sphenobasilar synchondrosis)

Ethmoid bone

Nasal bone

Occipital bone
Foramen magnum

Anterior atlanto-occiptal membrane

The spinal cord is continuous with the brainstem at the spinomedullary junction

Apical ligment of dens

Posterior tubercle of atlas

Membrana tectoria

Dura mater

Ligamentum nuchae

Anterior longitudinal ligament

Posterior longitudinal ligament

Spinal cord

Layers continue through the thoracic region

Spinal cord

Anterior longitudinal ligament

Spinous process

Interspinous ligament

Conus medullaris

Dura mater

Posterior longitudinal ligament

Lumbar cistern for cauda equina

Filum terminale internum

Sacrospinous tubercle

Sacral promontory

Sacral canal

Filum terminale externum

Anterior sacrococcygeal ligament

Deep posterior sacrococcygeal ligament

Sacral cornu

Coccyx

Pubic symphysis

Superior posterior sacrococcygeal ligament (completes sacral canal)

Genitourinary aperture

Perineal body

Anococcygeal ligament

Anal sphincter

This schematic illustration is not anatomically proportional but is produced to indicated tissue continuity.

Figure 3.1 Craniococcygeal Anatomy

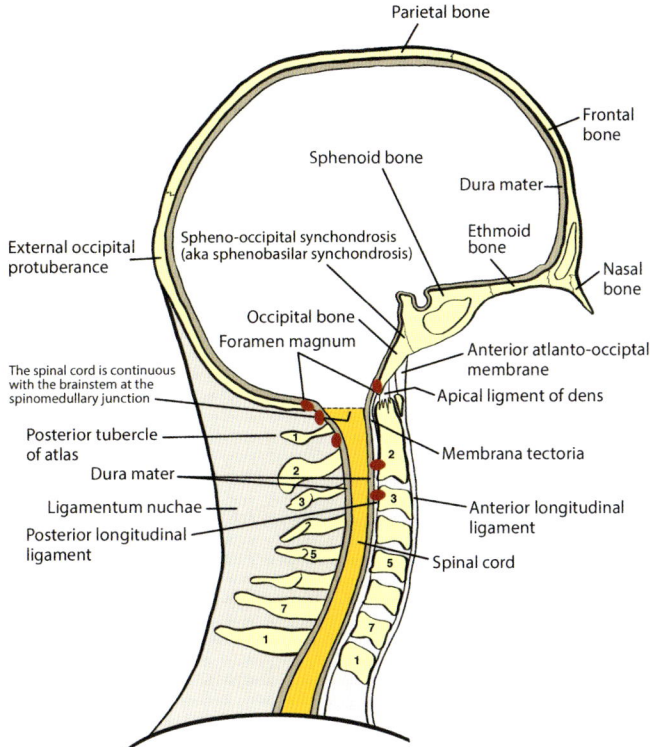

This schematic illustration is not anatomically proportional but is produced to indicated tissue continuity.

Figure 3.2 Craniococcygeal Anatomy, Upper

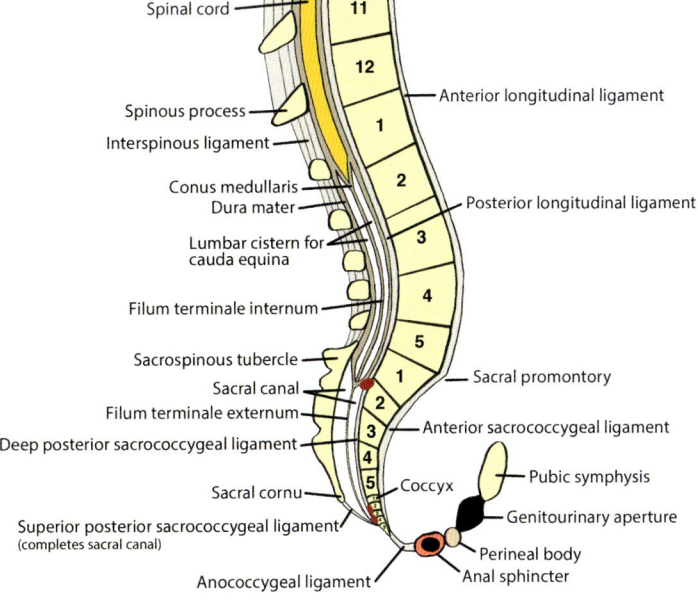

This schematic illustration is not anatomically proportional but is produced to indicated tissue continuity.

Figure 3.3 Craniococcygeal Anatomy, Lower

7. Anterior longitudinal ligament: Extends from the basilar part of the occipital bone to the anterior tubercle of C1 and the body of C2 and continues caudally attached to the anterior vertebral bodies and intervertebral discs of the cervical, thoracic, and lumbar vertebrae. Transitions to the anterior sacrococcygeal ligament at its attachments along the upper anterior aspect of the sacrum.

8. Posterior longitudinal ligament: Lies on the posterior surfaces of the vertebral bodies and intervertebral discs in the vertebral canal, attached between the body of C2 and the sacrum. It is continuous above with the membrana tectoria.

9. Membrana tectoria: Strong broad band that is the superior continuation of the posterior longitudinal ligament. Attaches to the posterior body of C2, capsule of the atlanto-occipital joint, and basilar part of the occipital bone and blends with the cranial dura mater above the foramen magnum.

10. Anterior and posterior sacrococcygeal ligaments: These are respectively continuous with the anterior and posterior longitudinal ligaments (see items 7 and 8).

    a. Anterior sacrococcygeal ligament (a.k.a. ventral sacrococcygeal ligament): Consists of irregular fibers that attach to the anterior surface of the sacrum and the first and second coccygeal vertebral bodies.

    b. Posterior sacrococcygeal ligament (a.k.a. dorsal sacrococcygeal ligament): Attaches to the posterior surface of the coccyx. Contains deep and superficial portions separated by the filum terminale externum.

        i. Superior posterior sacrococcygeal ligament: Extends from the margin of the sacral hiatus to the dorsal coccygeal surface, forming the roof of the lower sacral canal.

        ii. Deep posterior sacrococcygeal ligament: Is continuous with the posterior longitudinal ligament. It attaches from the back of the fifth sacral body to the dorsum of the coccyx and corresponds to the posterior longitudinal ligament.

11. Lateral sacrococcygeal ligament: On each side, the ligaments connect the coccygeal transverse processes to the inferolateral sacral angles.

12. Intercornual ligament: On each side, the ligaments connect the sacral and coccygeal cornua.

13. Sacrococcygeal fasciculi: Connect the sacral cornua to the coccygeal transverse processes.

14. Anococcygeal ligament: Layered musculotendinous ligament between the external anal sphincter and the coccyx.

15. Perineal body: An aggregation of fibromuscular tissue located in the midline at the junction between the anal and urogenital triangles, just anterior to the

external anal sphincter. It is attached to many structures in both the deep and superficial perineal spaces. Posteriorly, it merges with fibers from the external anal sphincter and the conjoint longitudinal coat. Superiorly, it is continuous with the rectovesical or rectovaginal septum, including fibers from levator ani (puboanalis or pubovaginalis). Anteriorly, it receives a contribution from the deep and superficial transverse perineal muscles and bulbospongiosus. The perineal body is continuous with the perineal membrane and the superficial perineal fascia. Since the latter runs forward into the skin of the perineum, the perineal body is tethered to the skin of the central perineum, which is often puckered over it. In males, this is continuous with the raphe of the scrotum. In females, the perineal body lies directly posterior to, and is attached to, the posterior commissure of the labia majora and the vaginal orifice. It has a fundamental role in the integrity of the pelvic floor, particularly in women. It can be compromised and rupture with vaginal birth, leading to widening and stretching of the levator ani muscle.

16. Levator ani: A broad muscular sheet of variable thickness attached to the internal surface of the pelvis along the condensation of the obturator fascia, which forms a large portion of the pelvic diaphragm. It is subdivided into named portions according to their attachments and the pelvic viscera to which they are related (pubococcygeus, iliococcygeus and puboanalis). Although they are often referred to as separate muscles, their boundaries are difficult to distinguish, and they have many similar physiological functions.

    a. Pubococcygeus: Arises from the posterior aspect of the pubis and inserts on the perineal body and anorectal junction.

        i. Males: Forms part of the urethral sphincter complex (pubourethralis).

        ii. Females: Forms a sling around the posterior wall of the vagina (pubovaginalis).

    b. Iliococcygeus: Posterior to the pubococcygeus, it originates on the inner surface of the ischial spine. Attaches to tip of the sacrum and coccyx and converges to form a fibrous raphe posterior to the anorectal junction continuous with the fibroelastic anococcygeal ligament.

    c. Ischiococcygeus (a.k.a. coccygeus): Some of the fibers attach to the sacrum and coccyx. Remaining parts of the muscle also converge in the midline. May be completely tendinous rather than muscular. Apex of the muscle arises as a musculotendinous sheet attached to the pelvic surface and tip of the ischial spine. Base of the muscle attaches to the lateral margins of the coccyx and the fifth sacral segment.

17. Gluteus maximus: Origin includes the posterolateral surface of the sacrum and coccyx.

18. Internal and external anal sphincters: Tonic state of contraction constricts the anal canal to prevent defecation. Both sphincters relax to allow defecation.

    a. External anal sphincter is attached to the perineal body anteriorly and to the anococcygeal ligament posteriorly. The most proximal fibers blend with the inferior medial fibers of puboanalis and attach to the anococcygeal raphe posteriorly and superficial transverse perineal muscle anteriorly.

    b. Internal anal sphincter is created by aggregated fibers surrounding the anal canal and is the thickened terminal part of the inner circular muscle of the large intestine. Begins at the anorectal junction and ends proximal to the anal orifice.

19. Conus medullaris: Distal end of the spinal cord, more commonly located at the level of the first lumbar vertebra. The pia mater here is continuous with the filum terminale below.

20. Filum terminale: Thin strand of connective tissue that extends from the conus medullaris and connects the spinal cord to the dorsum of the coccyx. Superiorly, it is continuous with the pia mater of the spinal cord.

    a. Filum terminale internum: Originates from the caudal portion of the conus medullaris, continuous within extensions of the dural and arachnoid meninges, and reaches the caudal border of the second sacral vertebra. Is approximately 15 cm in length and is continuous with the pia mater of the conus medullaris above.

    b. Filum terminale externum: Runs between the deep and superficial portions of the posterior sacrococcygeal ligament. Blends with the investing dura mater to attach with the periosteum of the posterior surface of the coccyx. Is approximately 5 cm in length.

21. Spinal dura mater: Forms a tube connecting the sacrococcygeal skeleton to the cranial skeleton.

    a. Superior attachments: foramen magnum, ligamentum nuchae at the level of the atlanto-occipital and atlantoaxial joints, and posterior bodies of C2 and C3.

    b. Midsubstance attachments: posterior longitudinal ligament of the lower vertebral column.

    c. Inferior attachments: filum terminale externum and the posterior surface of the coccyx.

22. Ganglion impar (a.k.a. coccygeal, sacrococcygeal, or Walther's ganglion): The terminal ganglion of the sympathetic trunks, formed by the confluence of the inferior right and left sympathetic trunks. Located close to the midline anywhere from the anterior inferior surface of the sacrococcygeal junction to the lower coccygeal vertebral bodies. This is the only place in the body where the right and left sympathetic trunks unite.

A Summary of the Anatomical Continuity from Cranium to Coccygeal Region

The anatomical relationship supporting the cranial to sacrococcygeal continuity is discussed as a three-segment model from anterior to posterior (Figure 3.4).

1. **Anterior:** The anterior atlanto-occipital membrane extends between the anterior margin of the foramen magnum and the upper border of the anterior arch of C1 and blends inferiorly with the anterior longitudinal ligament, which attaches to C1, C2, anterior vertebral bodies, and the intervertebral discs of the remaining cervical, thoracic, and lumbar vertebrae, and continues as the the anterior sacrococcygeal ligament attached to the anterior of the sacrum and coccyx.

2. **Middle:** The membrana tectoria originates on the base of the occiput and blends with the cranial dura mater and with the posterior longitudinal ligament that attaches to C2, posterior vertebral bodies, and the intervertebral discs of the remaining cervical, thoracic, and lumbar vertebrae; the deep posterior sacrococcygeal ligament which passes from the back of the fifth sacral vertebral body to the dorsum of the coccyx and corresponds to the posterior longitudinal ligament.

3. **Posterior:** Spinal dura mater attachments to foramen magnum, ligamentum nuchae, posterior bodies of C2 and C3 vertebrae, posterior longitudinal ligament of the lower vertebral column, filum terminale internum, filum terminale externum, and posterior surface of the coccyx (Standring 2020).

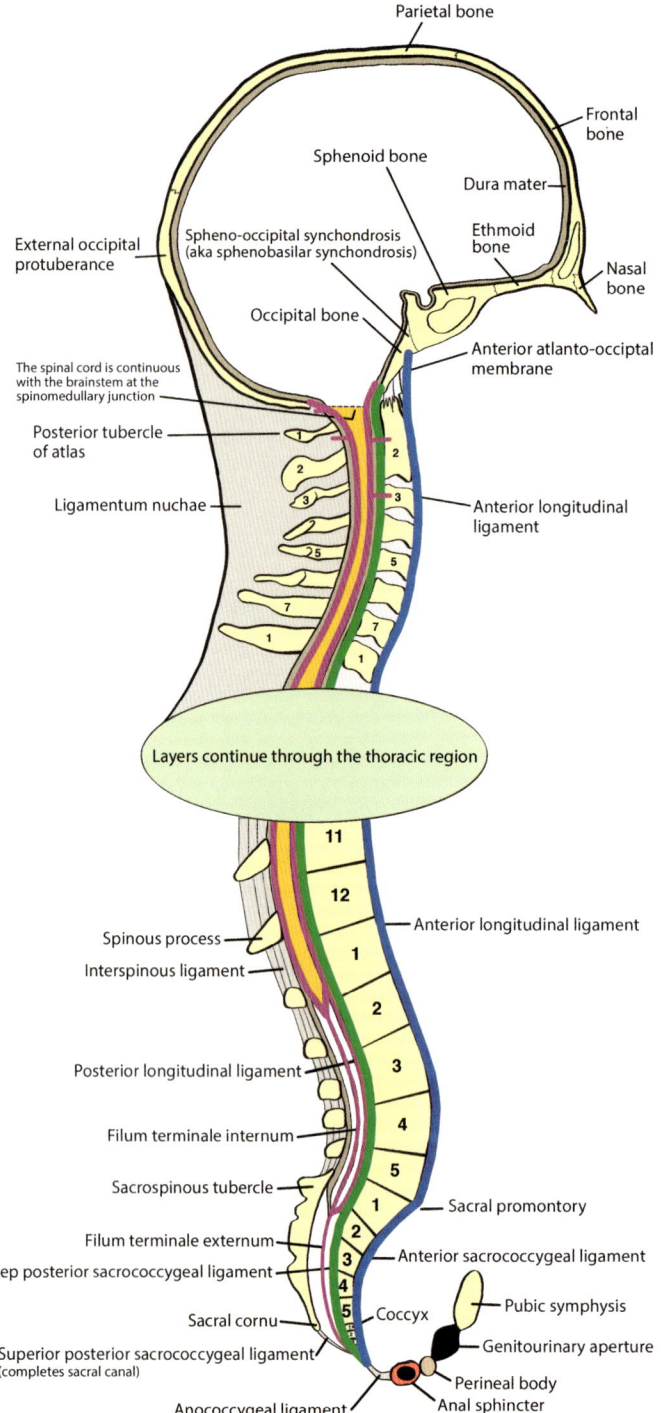

This schematic illustration is not anatomically proportional but is produced to indicated tissue continuity.

Figure 3.4 Craniococcygeal Continuity. The three layers of cranial to caudal continuity: posterior layer in pink, middle in green, anterior in blue.

Pretreatment Evaluation

History often supports a diagnosis of sacrococcygeal somatic dysfunction. This may include traumatic injury resulting from a fall, skiing, snowboarding, horseback riding, a kick to the tailbone, or a painful/traumatic birth.

Prior to examination, physician should inform the patient of palpation and evaluation of sacrococcygeal areas and obtain consent to evaluate. Physician should take appropriate steps to ensure patient safety, comfort, and modesty as much as possible during the exam.

Patient position: Prone. Physician palpates the following bony and soft tissue structures, evaluating for tenderness, asymmetry, restrictions, and tissue texture changes of the following structures:

1. Lateral surface of the sacrum and coccyx—attachments of levator ani muscle, gluteus maximus, sacrotuberous and sacrospinous ligaments: Thumb pads contact the soft tissue immediately lateral to sacrum and coccyx. Apply pressure from lateral to medial until detecting firm bony resistance. Evaluate for rotation and side-bending at the sacrococcygeal junction and coccygeal segments. Note tenderness or structural asymmetry.

2. Midline sacrum from superior to inferior: Palpate for tenderness and/or joint laxity of the sacrococcygeal junction. Continue careful palpation down each segment of the coccyx inferiorly until the inferior-most surface of the coccyx is reached. Note tenderness or displacement in the coronal, sagittal, and transverse planes.

3. Sacrococcygeal junction: Evaluate right and left sides simultaneously using thumb pads. Note tenderness or displacement.

   a. Inferior sacrum between sacral ala and superior coccyx

   b. Horizontal axis of sacrococcygeal junction

   c. Lateral surface of first coccygeal segment

   d. Inferior surface of first coccygeal segment

Most Common Treatment Indications

1. Tenderness to palpation reproducing the patient's pain.

2. Local pain to palpation out of proportion to patient's or physician's expectations with asymmetry or restricted range of motion.

Informed Consent and Documentation

Prior to any internal procedure, informed verbal consent must be obtained directly from the adult patient and/or responsible party. Informed consent is the dialogue between patient and physician that includes a discussion and/or assessment of each of the following (Braddock et al. 1997; Cordasco 2013):

1. The patient's role in the decision-making process.

2. Clinical issue.

3. Suggested treatment.

4. Option for no treatment and/or alternative treatments.

5. Potential risks and benefits of recommended treatment and alternative treatments.

6. Related uncertainties.

7. Patient's understanding of the information.

8. Obtaining the patient's preference and consent.

Discussion should also include a detailed review of the internal procedure and goals of therapy. Verbal consent should take place in the presence of a chaperone and family member, if present. If the practice has a system in place for the chaperone to document within the chart, it is suggested for the chaperone to document that (1) they witnessed informed consent by the patient and (2) they chaperoned the entire duration of the internal procedure. If the patient is a minor, physician should refer to state laws and obtain informed consent accordingly. The physician should document that informed consent was obtained, including detailed review of internal procedure, goals of therapy, alternatives, potential risks and benefits, and medical necessity. Documentation should also include if there were any complications, such as bleeding or excessive pain, and patient outcome. The subjective section should support the indications for the exam and treatment. The objective section should support the reason for treatment.

Clinical Procedure

Treatment should ensure patient safety, comfort, and modesty as much as possible. Provide the patient with the opportunity to use the restroom prior to the procedure. The principles of Long Lever Technique apply throughout, with a final goal of treating barriers, improving biomechanics, and detecting the primary respiratory mechanism integrated with the surrounding structures.

Supplies

1. Gloves
2. Lubricant
3. Gauze or similar cleaning wipe
4. Wastebasket

Position

Patient position

    a. Parts 1 and 3: Prone. Chest and head resting against the table (Figure 3.5).

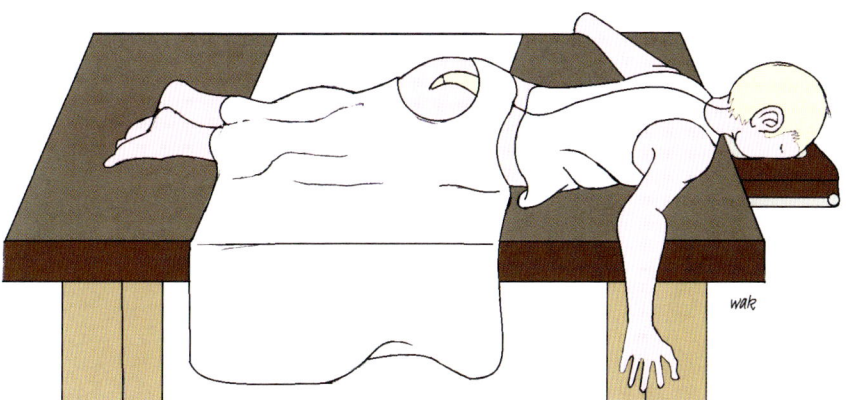

Figure 3.5 Prone position. Patient face down, chest resting on table.

  b. Part 2: Prone-propped, a.k.a. sphinx position (Figure 3.6).

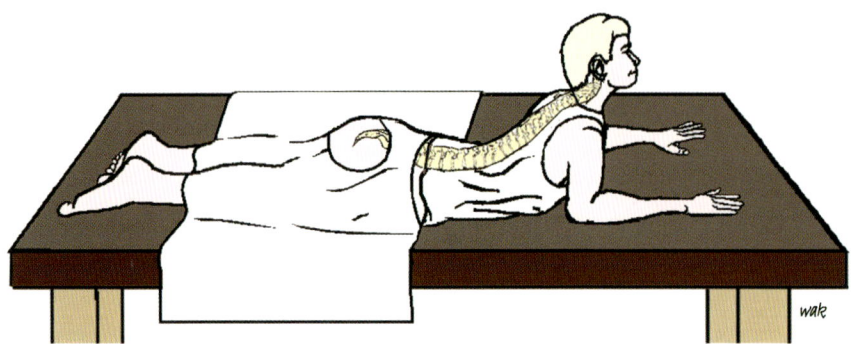

Figure 3.6 Prone-propped, a.k.a. sphinx position. Patient is prone, with lumbar hyperextension, resting on elbows. Chest and head are lifted as tolerated.

2. Physician position: To the side of patient, facing the patient's head. Physician's dominant hand should be closest to the patient (i.e., a right-handed physician will stand at the left side of the patient's prone body).

Part 1: Soft Tissue

1. Patient position: Prone. Chest and head resting against the table (Figure 3.5).

2. Physician gently inserts lubricated gloved index finger into patient's anus.

3. With internal index finger and external thumb contacting the soft tissue structures, evaluate for tenderness, restrictions, and increased or decreased tone of the following soft tissue structures distal to the coccyx and surrounding the sacrococcygeal joint:

  a. Anococcygeal ligament

  b. Levator ani

    i. Pubococcygeus

    ii. Iliococcygeus

    iii. Ischiococcygeus

  c. External and internal anal sphincters

4. Treat if there is tenderness or resistance in soft tissue range of motion.

*Note: For this part, I more commonly utilize indirect methods, such as myofascial release, balanced ligamentous tension, ligamentous articular strain, facilitated positional release, exaggerated method, or functional technique (see **Glossary of Osteopathic Terminology** or **Foundations of Osteopathic Medicine**).*

Part 2: Bony and Ligamentous Structures

Transition from Part 1 to Part 2 of treatment is seamless, with physician's finger remaining transrectal.

1. Patient position: Prone-propped, a.k.a. sphinx position (Figure 3.6). Patient is prone, with lumbar hyperextension, resting on elbows. Chest and head are not resting on the treatment table.

2. Physician's transrectal index finger and external thumb contact the inferior tip of the coccyx (Figure 3.7).

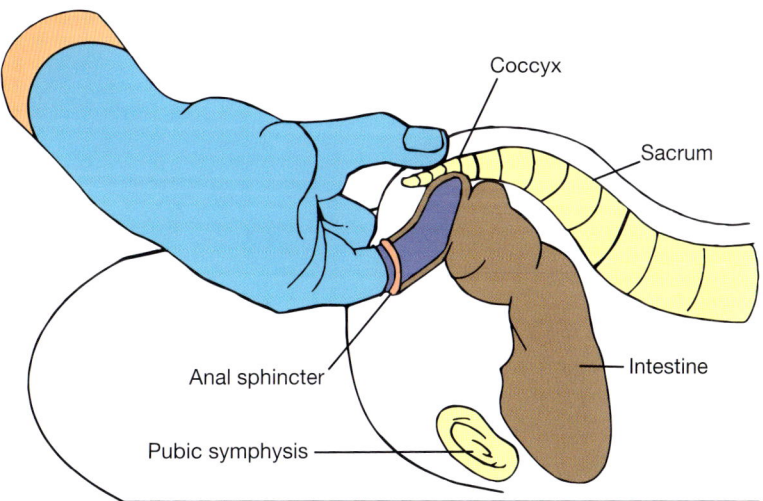

Figure 3.7 Transrectal finger contacting anterior sacrococcygeal surface while external thumb contacting posterior surface.

3. Evaluate for tenderness or restrictions of the following:

   a. Distal coccygeal tip

   b. Each coccygeal segment, including attachments at the transverse processes of the first coccygeal segment

   c. Sacrococcygeal junction

   d. Inferior sacrum

   e. Lateral sacrococcygeal ligaments

   f. Anterior and posterior sacrococcygeal ligaments

4. Transrectal index finger and external thumb are used to identify and treat sites of tenderness or restricted range of motion with simultaneous patient assistance.

   a. Physician localizes tender area and/or sites of restriction between thumb and index finger. Physician engages the sacrococcygeal barrier.

   b. Patient is asked to slowly move their head and neck in each plane of motion to localize to the site of dysfunction.

   c. Long lever: Patient's head. Patient actively assists in treatment by moving their head and neck slowly toward and away from the barrier in all three planes of motion (Figure 3.8).

     i. Flexion/extension

    ii. Rotation right and left

   iii. Sidebending right and left

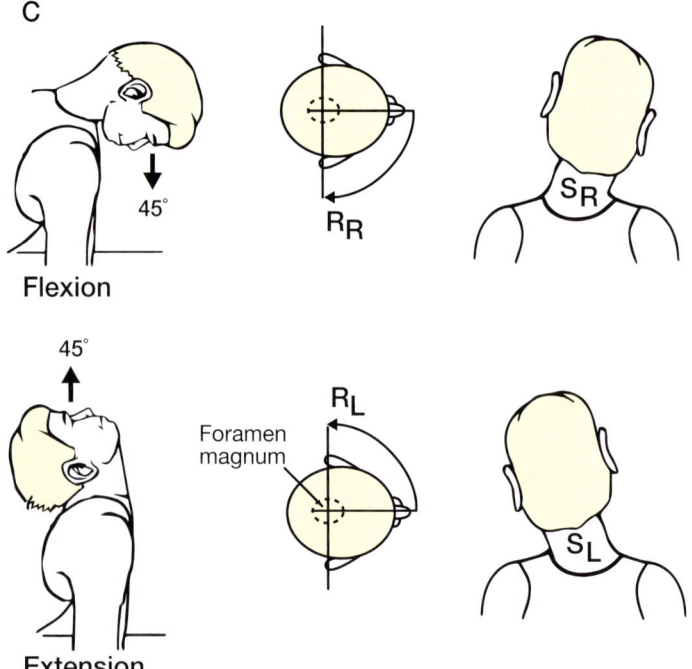

Figure 3.8 Three planes of cervical motion, including flexion/extension, rotation, and sidebending.

d. Physician maintains balanced tension until improvement in sacrococcygeal somatic dysfunction is detected. Patient's head movement at the direction of the physician helps the physician maintain the dysfunction at the barrier while treatment is in process.

e. For best patient comfort, educate the patient to slowly move their head in the direction of the barrier without aggressively trying to push through it. When the patient feels tightening and resistance in either their head, neck, or sacrococcygeal areas, the patient backs off about 30 degrees before repeating head and neck motion toward the barrier. Range of motion increases in the direction of the barrier with each attempt, until the final barrier is passed. This often takes a few attempts by the patient, moving toward and away from the barrier. Instruction may be as follows: "Gently move your head toward the front door of the barrier without going through it. Then move your head 30 degrees in the opposite direction. Slowly repeat."

f. Physician constantly maintains localized balanced tension at the sacrococcygeal dysfunction. Monitor for patient's movements, and provide feedback to patient, to best localize directions of patient's movements, pace, and force.

g. Treat tender and restricted areas.

Part 3: Soft Tissue

1. Patient position: Prone. Chest and head resting against the table (Figure 3.5).

2. Physician's transrectal index finger and extrarectal thumb contact the following soft tissue structures and evaluate for tenderness or restrictions:

    a. Midsubstance and pelvic attachments of sacrotuberous and sacrospinous ligaments

    b. Levator ani muscle

    c. Anococcygeal ligament

3. Treat if there is tenderness or resistance in soft tissue range of motion.

*Note: For this part, I more commonly utilize indirect methods, such as myofascial release, balanced ligamentous tension, ligamentous articular strain, facilitated positional release, exaggerated method, or functional technique (see **Glossary of Osteopathic Terminology** or **Foundations of Osteopathic Medicine**).*

Part 4: Post-Treatment

Provide patient with cleaning materials and wastebasket. Allow patient to clean, dress, and use restroom as needed.

Post-Treatment Evaluation

Reassess findings from pretreatment evaluation. Compare for tissue texture changes, asymmetry, restrictions, and tenderness. Ask patient to subjectively assess pain while seated, standing, and lying down. A case report and a case series both suggest that changes in seated pain scores are most reflective of patient outcome.

Post-Treatment Recommendations

Encourage the patient to go for a brief walk as tolerated. Avoid sitting on hard surfaces or for prolonged periods for the first 48 hours. Avoid sexual activity for 24 hours. Avoid painful activities. Consider individualized rehabilitative exercises.

Potential Side Effects

Menstrual irregularity, including menorrhagia and menometrorrhagia, often resolve within one to two cycles. Bowel movement consistency and frequency may take one to two weeks to normalize. Perirectal tissue soreness from transrectal manipulation often resolves within several days post-procedure.

Potential Treatment Benefits

During the treatment, a majority of patients can recognize a craniosacral connection when moving their head and neck while the physician localizes the sacrococcygeal restrictions. In addition to pain reduction post-treatment, some patients have noted improvements of the following: restlessness, pressured speech, emotional lability, verbal outbursts, crying, unusual anger, constipation, hemorrhoids, and headaches. The physiological causes for all of these improvements are not directly understood, but they are likely associated with decreased pain and reduced mechanical stress on soft tissue, nerves, and bony structures.

Acknowledgments

A sincere thank you to the following people for their support and participation: illustrators William Kuchera, DO, FAAO, Dist. and Zac Miller; reviewer of craniococcygeal anatomical relationships by Susan Standring, PhD, DSc, MBE, professor emeritus of anatomy, Department of Anatomy, King's College London, editor-in-chief of *Gray's Anatomy;* and Amy Fulcher, OMS3, for her assistance with the literature review and early communication with Dr. Standring.

References

Braddock, C. H., III, Fihn, S. D., Levinson, W., Jonsen, A. R., & Pearlman, R. A. (1997). How doctors and patients discuss routine clinical decisions. Informed decision making in the outpatient setting. *Journal of General Internal Medicine, 12*(6), 339–345.

Capar, B., Akpinar, N., Kutluay, E., Müjde, S., & Turan, A. (2007). Coccygectomy in patients with coccydynia. *Acta Orthopaedica et Traumatologica Turcica, 41*(4), 277–280.

Cordasco, K. (2013). Obtaining informed consent from patients: Brief update review. *Making Health Care Safer II: An Updated Critical Analysis of the Evidence for Patient Safety Practices.* Evidence Reports/Technology Assessments, No. 211 (March), Chapter 39. Rockville, MD: Agency for Healthcare Research and Quality (US). www.ncbi.nlm.nih.gov/books/NBK133402/.

Giusti, R. (Ed.). (2017). *Glossary of osteopathic terminology* (3rd ed.). Chevy Chase, MD: American Association of Colleges of Osteopathic Medicine.

Howard, P. D., Dolan, A. N., Falco, A. N., Holland, B. M., Wilkinson, C. F., & Zink, A. M. (2013). A comparison of conservative interventions and their effectiveness for coccydynia: A systematic review. *Journal of Manual & Manipulative Therapy, 21*(4), 213–219.

Kerr, E. E., Benson, D., & Schrot, R. J. (2011). Coccygectomy for chronic refractory coccygodynia: Clinical case series and literature review. *Journal of Neurosurgery: Spine, 14*(5), 654–663.

Lirette, L. S., Chaiban, G., Tolba, R., & Eissa, H. (2014). Coccydynia: An overview of the anatomy, etiology, and treatment of coccyx pain. *Ochsner Journal, 14*(1), 84–87.

Nathan, S. T., Fisher, B. E., & Roberts, C. S. (2010). Coccydynia: A review of pathoanatomy, aetiology, treatment and outcome. *Journal of Bone & Joint Surgery: British volume, 92*(12), 1622–1627.

Nourani, B., Gilbert, R., & Rabago, D. (2020). The treatment of coccydynia and headache with transrectal OMT: A case report. *Scholar: Pilot and Validation Studies, 1*(1), 14–18.

Patel, R., Appannagari, A., & Whang, P. G. (2008). Coccydynia. *Current Reviews in Musculoskeletal Medicine, 1*(3–4), 223–226.

Pennekamp, P. H., Kraft, C. N., Stütz, A., Wallny, T., Schmitt, O., & Diedrich, O. (2005). Coccygectomy for coccygodynia: Does pathogenesis matter? *Journal of Trauma, 59*(6), 1414–1419.

Schapiro, S. (1950). Low back and rectal pain from an orthopedic and proctologic viewpoint; with a review of 180 cases. *American Journal of Surgery, 79*(1), 117–128.

Seffinger, M. (2018). *Foundations of osteopathic medicine: Philosophy, science, clinical applications, and research.* Philadelphia: Wolters Kluwer.

Standring, S. (Ed.). (2020). *Gray's anatomy: The anatomical basis of clinical practice* (42nd ed.). Saint Louis, MO: Elsevier.

Thiele, G. H. (1963). Coccygodynia: Cause and treatment. *Diseases of the Colon & Rectum, 6,* 422–436.

Trollegaard, A. M., Aarby, N. S., & Hellberg, S. (2010). Coccygectomy: An effective treatment option for chronic coccydinia: Retrospective results in 41 consecutive patients. *Journal of Bone & Joint Surgery: British volume, 92*(2), 242–245.

PART 4

Integrating
Long Lever Techniques in Practice

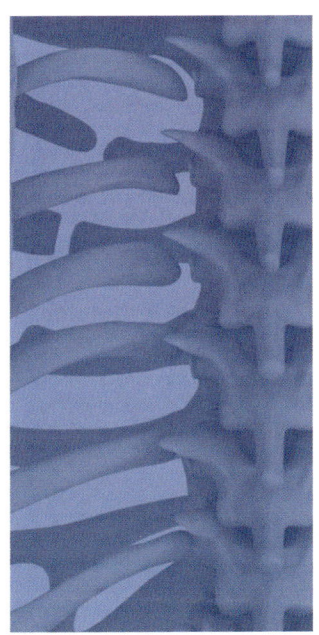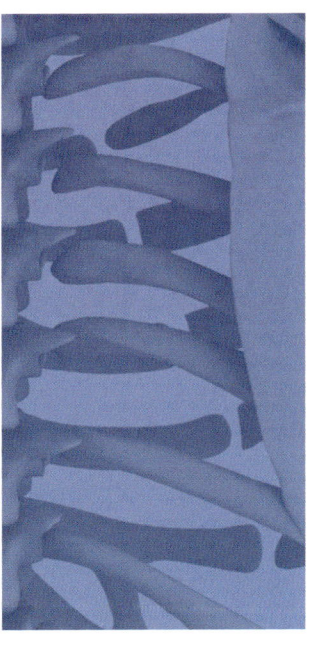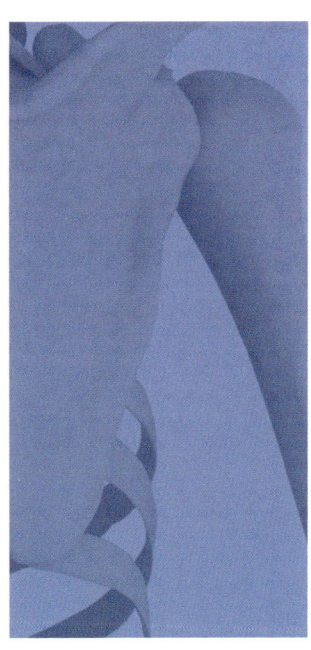

Osteopathic Beginnings

KENNETH LOSSING, DO

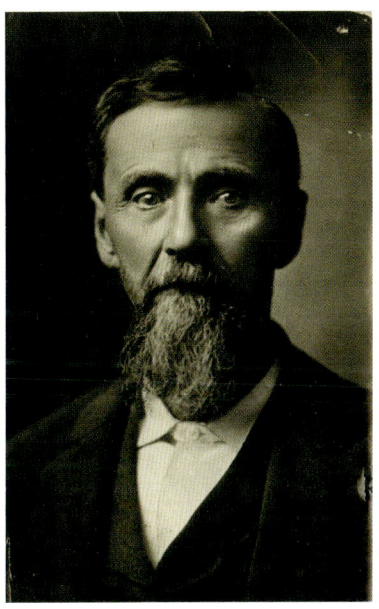

Andrew Taylor Still, DO
Founder of Osteopathy

In 1874, Andrew Taylor Still, MD, first conceived the ideas that became osteopathy (Still 1897) based on a few simple and profound ideas:

1. Mechanics are as important as chemistry. The function of any structure relies on both proper mechanical and biochemical processes, equally.

2. All body systems interact. The body works as an integrated whole, and all interrelations must be appreciated.

3. The body will function well if its mechanical processes proceed smoothly and properly.

Still claimed that palpable changes are found in any area of the body that is not working properly. The physical examination is important to understanding the patient's history and is a crucial component of formulating a diagnosis. An area is dysfunctional when life forces will not flow or properly regulate. A dysfunctional area reflects a problem but is not necessarily the root of the problem.

Diagnostics were virtually nonexistent in Still's time. The clinical diagnosis depended entirely on history and physical examination since these were the only diagnostic tools available. Still's respect for the history and physical examination was demonstrated in his curriculum. The American School of Osteopathy (ASO), founded in 1892, had nearly 500 hours during the first two years dedicated to physical examination and palpation. The length of physical examination education was a dramatic expansion over what was taught in medical schools of that time. The palpatory exam included bones, muscles, fascia, vasculature, nerves, and lymphatics. Physical evaluation included visual inspection and observation, auscultation, percussion, and palpation.

Still called his new science "osteopathy," meaning "to begin with the bones." To begin with the bones is to palpate the spine, ribs, extremities, etc., where a malposition might be found. This could be a complete or partial dislocation, or a mild restriction within the normal range, but the more a bone is displaced and limited in motion, the greater the effect on soft tissues, fascia, nerves, and circulation.

Mobility is motion caused by a secondary source, e.g., respiration. Localized restriction of motion can adversely affect the mobility of the entire body. Such dysfunction may be called a key lesion or dysfunction. Proper treatment of a key lesion can benefit the adjacent region or the entire body.

There are two basic types of dysfunction: anatomical and functional. Anatomical dysfunction is when a structure is broken, worn out, or torn. These may be seen radiologically, as with severe osteoarthritis, herniated discs, or ligamentous tears. Functional dysfunctions, or somatic dysfunctions, do not manifest with imaging. Somatic dysfunction is identified by skilled palpation. Palpable changes may include asymmetry, lack of motion, tissue texture and temperature changes relative to the surrounding area, and decreased flow when palpating the vascular or lymphatic structures. Fortunately, even anatomical dysfunctions have a functional component and therefore may, in part, improve with treatment.

Still taught anatomy and principles but very little technique. He did not want students copying him without understanding the body and its physiology. The few techniques he did write about were in *Osteopathy, Research and Practice* (Still 1910) and were only vague descriptions.

One approach that Still taught was the long lever principle, using lever and fulcrum to mobilize an area of somatic dysfunction. The force applied to one lever arm over a fulcrum moves the load (dysfunction). The longer the distance between applied force and fulcrum and the closer the fulcrum is to the load, the less force is required to move the load. This force can be applied one time or multiple times.

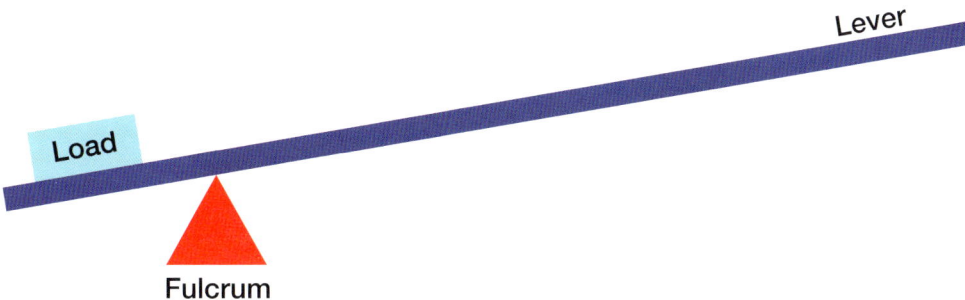

Although Still did not write much about his techniques, many of his students did. The first of Still's students to publish a book about his manipulative techniques was Elmer Barber, DO, who wrote *Osteopathy: The New Science of Healing* (1896) and later *Osteopathy Complete* (1898). The books were primarily Barber's class notes as a student. Some of the approaches detailed in Barber's books included soft tissue, visceral, and lymphatic. He described techniques using the physician's knees as long levers to articulate the spinal joints.

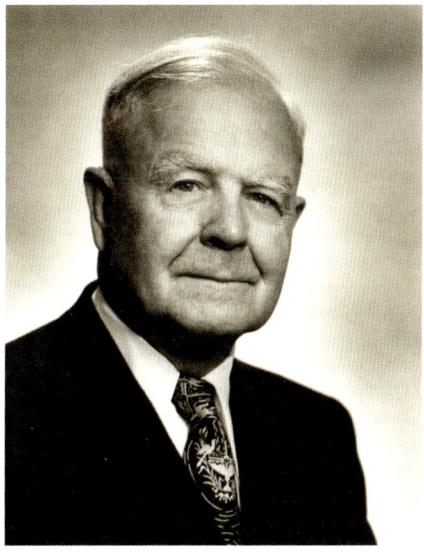

William Garner Sutherland, DO

In 1900, William Garner Sutherland was a student at the American School of Osteopathy (now called A.T. Still University). He walked by a Beauchene disarticulated skull in a hallway. The thought struck him that the sphenosquamosal sutures were beveled, like the gills of a fish. Perhaps it was some sort of breathing system requiring motion between the bevels? The thought haunted him, as he was taught that all sutures were fused in the adult and, thus, immovable.

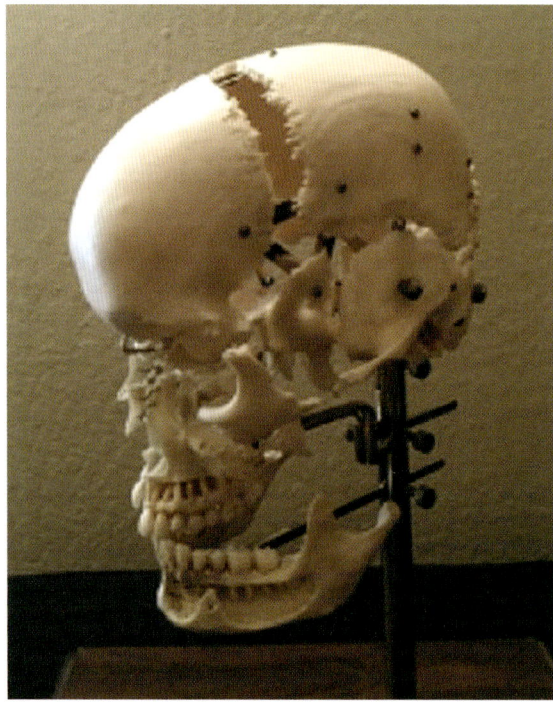

Beauchene skull

Over the next few years, Sutherland used his jackknife on his human cadaver skull, "Mike," to slowly disarticulate the sutures. Though not easily separated, they did come apart. Determining that they could and were meant to move, he then wondered what moves them and why? Sutherland also wondered if there were health/disease implications with restricted sutures. Palpating the heads of patients, he noticed they were often asymmetrical and even slightly pliable. Sutherland reasoned that, similar to the spine and extremities, sutures may also have articular patterns or strains that produce consequences to health. In order to understand what these were, he devised a system of straps and pads to reproduce them and to see if they had any ill effects on him. They did. His wife reported finding him nearly unconscious once and unable to move.

With time, and trial and error, Sutherland noticed that if he mobilized stuck sutures, he could feel a fluid-like motion consisting of expansion and contraction corresponding to the thoracic respiratory rate and movement of the respiratory diaphragm. Then, by mobilizing spinal articular strains, including the sacrum, the cranial motion improved with each respiratory cycle. This fluid motion also moved at a similar rate to thoracic respiration.

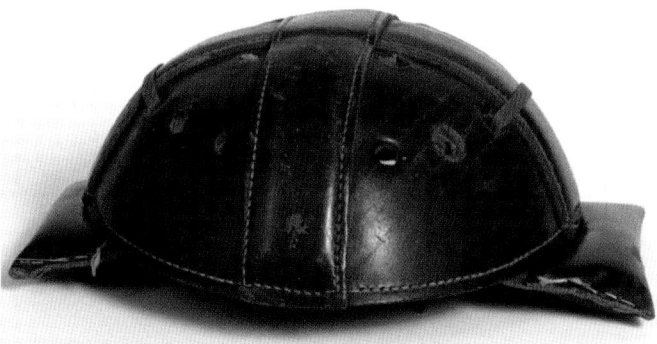

Dr. Sutherland used the device for experimentation on his own head during his early research. Tourniquets were passed through the holes and, together with side appendages, created compression to counteract expansions associated with sinus pathology, migraine, and other conditions. The original version was made from the upper part of a contemporary football helmet.

By the mid-1930s Sutherland having determined that his ideas were clinically useful, started to publish his ideas under the pen name "Blunt Bone Bill." With hardly a response from the osteopathic profession, in 1939 he published *The Cranial Bowl,* to declare his findings up to that point, presenting: the possible motions available in the head; that cerebrospinal fluid (CSF) fluctuated; what kinds of problems specific blows to the head created; and how to diagnose and treat those traumatic strains. Here Sutherland first mentioned the "primary respiratory mechanism," noticing the thoracic respiratory rate followed the primary respiratory rate.

Around 1939 Sutherland attended the American Osteopathic Association Convention, where two of the leaders of the osteopathic profession, George Northup and Perrin Wilson, became interested in his ideas. Northup, Wilson, Beryl Arbuckle, and a few other DOs would meet in Sutherland's home in St. Peter, Minnesota, to learn Sutherland's new approaches. In 1943 Arthur Becker, dean of the Des Moines school, invited Sutherland to teach a course at the university. Beryl Arbuckle was among the table trainers, and Becker's sons, Rollin and Alan, attended the class.

At this point, they were palpating skulls to find asymmetries, including motion testing the bones through their range of motion to identify areas of restriction. Through this, they noted that the majority of the strain patterns were caused by peripheral suture restrictions, not the sphenobasilar synchondrosis (SBS). Although true SBS strains do exist, they are most often caused by trauma during childhood, such as birth trauma, while the bones are still more flexible.

Around 1945 Sutherland included the direction of fluid for both diagnosis and treatment. Treatment was done with one hand placed with a finger on either side of the suture and the fingers tractioning laterally. The other hand produced a CSF wave directed toward the suture with a pointed finger from the opposite side of the head. The resulting waves were monitored to see if they would bounce back, like sonar, thus indicating bony or sutural restriction. The waves were continued until the area softened and the waves washed through the restriction, resulting in a softening of the suture.

Sutherland taught cranial motion testing until about 1948. At the time, the predominant spinal and extremity treatments taught in osteopathic schools were high-velocity, low-amplitude (HVLA) techniques. Almost no one taught the gentler exaggeration techniques Sutherland had been taught by Still. Consequently, the tactile skills of newer osteopathic students and physicians were unrefined. This was apparent at courses where students using too much force caused headaches and other undesired side effects. Sutherland changed cranial motion testing to initiation of motion, letting momentum and the fluid take the bone as far as it would go. This is only a fraction of the motion found by motion testing and, consequently, is less accurate.

The primary respiratory mechanism consists of the fluctuation of the cerebrospinal fluid, the mobility of the reciprocal tension membrane, the motility of the neural tube, the articular mobility of the sacrum between the ilia, and the articular mobility of the cranial bones. In 1949, Sutherland started talking about the fluid in the fluid, the potency, the force that drives the ocean tide, and the fluid motion in the central nervous system.

During his lifetime, Sutherland never talked about rates, except the respiratory rate. Drs. John and Rachel Woods, both students of Sutherland, checked the heads of 102 psychiatric patients and 62 control subjects at the Still-Hildreth Hospital (Woods and Woods 1961). The rhythmic cranial expansion and contraction of the psychiatric patients was much slower (6.7 cycles per minute) than the control group (12.47 cycles per minute). They called the cranial rate the cranial rhythmic impulse, or CRI. At nearly this same time, Dr. Rollin Becker found the average healthy individual to have a similar rate of 8–12 cycles per minute. Becker also observed a decreased rate during treatment to about 2.5 cycles per minute and sometimes even slower to 6 cycles per 10 minutes, which he called the long tide.

A neutral point, or still point, achieved during a treatment may rebalance the autonomic nervous system. It is similar in concept to rebooting a computer. The sympathetics, which commonly dominate, equilibrate with the parasympathetics. Often, when this happens, patients may relax or even fall asleep. This phenomenon is observed when doing breathing exercises to improve heart rate variability.

In the last few years of his life, Sutherland stressed using inherent forces of motility to treat strains. He spent more than fifty years treating sutural restrictions as articular membranous strains, normalizing mobility, and only then was able to achieve doing that with inherent motion. Though he did not write about this, it appears that Sutherland taught at least a few of his students how to palpate the PRM throughout the body, and to use it to treat the extremities and spine. This is how his student Anne Wales taught her students. Unfortunately, this was not recorded in any texts.

References

Barber, E. (1896). *Osteopathy: The new science of healing.* Kansas City, MO: Hudson-Kimberly Publishing.

Barber, E. (1898). *Osteopathy complete.* Kansas City, MO: Hudson-Kimberly Publishing.

Lippincott, R. C., & Lippincott, H. A. (1943). *A manual of cranial technique.* Ann Arbor, MI: Edward Brothers.

Magoun, H. (1951). *Osteopathy in the cranial field* (1st ed.). Kirksville, MO: Journal Printing Company.

McManis, V. J. (1915). *McManis table: Detailed information.* Dayton, OH: McManis Table Company.

Missouri Digital Heritage, Museum of Osteopathic Medicine, A.T. Still Collection. Images and descriptions reprinted with permission. https://www.atsu.edu/museum-of-osteopathic-medicine/a-t-still-papers-american-school-of-osteopathy-aso

Personal communications: Susie Clark-Wismer, DO; Anne Wales, DO; Robert Fulford, DO; Thomas Schooley, DO; Viola Frymann, DO; Herb Miller, DO; Alan Becker, DO; Stefan Hagopian, DO; Brian Degenhardt, DO.

Simel, D. L., & Drummond, R. (Eds.). (2009). *The rational clinical examination.* New York: McGraw-Hill.

Still, A.T. (1897). *Autobiography of Andrew T. Still.* Kirksville, MO: A.T. Still.

Still, A.T. (1910). *Osteopathy, research and practice.* Kirksville, MO: A.T. Still.

Strand, A., & Whales, A. (Eds.). (1967). *Contributions of thought: Collected writings of William Garner Sutherland.* Sutherland Cranial Teaching Foundation.

Sutherland, A. (1962). *With thinking fingers.* Kansas City, MO: Cranial Academy.

Sutherland Memorial Library, Texas College of Osteopathic Medicine (TCOM).

Sutherland, W.G. (1939). *The cranial bowl.* Mankato, MN: Free Press Company.

Sutherland, W.G. (1990). *Teachings in the science of osteopathy.* (A. Wales, Ed.). Fort Worth, TX: Rudra Press.

Woods, R. H., & Woods, J. M. (1961). A physical finding related to psychiatric disorders. *Journal of the American Osteopathic Association, 60*(12): 988–993. https://ostemed-dr.contentdm.oclc.org/digital/collection/myfirst/id/13044/.

Yamada, T. (Ed.). (1999). *Yamada's textbook of gastroenterology* (3rd ed.). Philadelphia: Lippincott Williams & Wilkins.

The Quantum of Healing: Interexaminer Reliability

CHARLIE BECK, DO, FAAO

In March 2010, an interesting experiment took place at the American Academy of Osteopathy's (AAO) Annual Convocation. The experiment started with Dr. Ed Stiles, DO, FAAO, Dist., wishing to observe and understand the treatment given to a patient by Paul Hume, ND, DO, of New Zealand. A group of six physicians, all former students or residents of Dr. Stiles, were on hand to observe and participate in the experiment. Drs. Stiles and Hume agreed that both would evaluate the patient, one would treat any given somatic dysfunction, and then both would check the results.

The group was there to observe the interaction. Some of those in the group noticed that when Dr. Stiles approached the patient, the patient's left innominate moved cephalad. When Stiles moved away, the innominate moved back to its original position. When Dr. Hume approached the patient, it was noted that the right innominate moved cephalad. When Hume moved away, it again returned to its original position. The group paused the treatment to discuss the findings. The process was repeated, with the same observations each of the three times it was repeated.

In medical school, we are taught that innominate findings are static when making accurate diagnoses. It is how we are tested in school and the basis upon which we treat patients. What happened before us defied this completely. The group continued observing as Drs. Hume and Stiles approached from the head, then from the feet, asking questions as they went along to explain the variances in findings between the two examiners. The group discovered the patient's body consistently presented differently to each examiner. When Dr. Stiles approached the patient, the patient's body manifested in one way, whereas when Dr. Hume approached the patient, the patient's dysfunction manifested differently irrespective of the examiner's physical approach to the patient.

In quantum physics, a quantum is the smallest unit of energy, and when quanta interact, they influence each other. Each examiner presents quanta of life experiences, including past training, belief systems, previous patient encounters, etc. These factors come into play each time an examiner approaches a patient.

The patient, a quantum of experience as well, interacts and responds accordingly, producing different presentations for each examiner. It is as though the patient's body changes as the practitioner approaches, in order to align with the practitioner's quanta, i.e., training and skill. Thus, the patient's body apparently adapts to how the practitioner can best treat it.

Dr. Hume's approach appeared to be cerebral, using knowledge of anatomy, movement patterns, etc., to guide his palpation, and so he named the anatomy as he treated. Dr. Stiles let his palpation guide him through the anatomy and movement patterns. He palpated motion to identify the patient's anatomy.

Their differences demonstrate the two predominant patterns of teaching in osteopathy. Hume was taught to study anatomy first and then let the knowledge of that anatomy guide palpation. This style predominates when teaching technique-based treatment. Stiles focuses on the palpatory experience to guide the learning of anatomy. This predominates with principle-based teaching.

What the group observed between Stiles and Hume was that Stiles' approach to treatment involved using more of his heart and intuition to assess, whereas Hume primarily used his mind. Stiles relied on touching the patient to paint the picture of the anatomy under his hands. On the other hand, Hume relied on his knowledge of anatomy to paint the picture of what his hands were feeling. His knowledge of anatomy guided his touch and assessment. Stiles let his hands bring the anatomy to mind, whereas Hume used his knowledge of the anatomical structures to guide his hands.

This difference has led to much discussion and a fair amount of evaluation of how practitioners palpate. Some osteopaths lead with their hands to explore the anatomy, and others use anatomical knowledge to guide their palpation. Because this realization leads to at least two ways to explore anatomy, the question has been raised about why these two different methods of evaluation have not been presented in tandem in osteopathic teaching thus far. The typical osteopathic education is set up for auditory and visual learners. Stiles has observed in his teaching career that many of the best manipulators are kinesthetic learners. Interestingly enough, these often also play a musical instrument. Combining these learning styles—auditory, visual, and kinesthetic—with an osteopathic curriculum could introduce anatomy and palpation in a way that more students could understand and successfully utilize.

As strange as these realizations may seem, they do explain why issues with interexaminer reliability exist within osteopathy. With each osteopath bringing quanta that interact with and produce patient responses, unless educators can identify and teach students to identify these influences, similarity in assessment will not be consistent, and students will be confused over what is actually happening when they touch a patient.

The group witnessed two practitioners coming up with diagnoses that seldom agreed. Each rendered a treatment, but not where the other would have. Both achieved similar results, though Stiles would have finished sooner than Hume. Stiles noted a slowed response to treatment, indicating maximal improvement. Stiles has often wished he could test when to stop treatment (or in what order to treat) by taking a patient back to the beginning after treatment had completed, to try again using a different sequence or method. Were this possible, interexaminer issues could be sorted out more easily.

At the AAO Convocation in Dallas, Texas, in March 2018, Stiles met with Richard Huff, DO, and a similar group of observers with a new patient to repeat a similar experiment. Palpating the patient, Stiles and Huff identified what each considered the key area or problem. After questioning and observing the two practitioners, the observers concluded that each practitioner was palpating a different layer of anatomy. Stiles's attention was on the fascial layer; Huff's was on the ligamentous. Only through their interaction did each realize they were doing something different from the other. More questions led to the discovery that each was placing forces (loading) into the body differently when palpating.

Huff induced tension into the body to identify ligamentous response to his tissue loading. Stiles loaded the fascial system to assess its response to the forces placed upon it. Each practitioner was certain he was palpating identically to the other. Each was sure he had identified the correct key lesion. The group observed the treatment of the patient as each practitioner made a reassessment after a portion of the treatment was rendered. More interexaminer reliability issues were noted. Each practitioner was certain he was doing the same thing as the other, but observations, comments, and questions of the group teased out the differences.

The conclusions from this experiment were compared to those of the 2010 experiment, and in doing so the observers learned something about themselves. Each osteopathic school presumably teaches students how to determine their dominant eye. What the groups observed in testing each other is that, while knowing one's dominant eye is important, knowing how that affects the palpatory experience of each is far more important. We learn in our formal education how each of us has preferential eye dominance. This can vary with arms extended versus arms bent. Some practitioners can have a mixture (one eye dominant with arms extended, and the other eye dominant with arms bent). This is called mixed eye dominance. For some, eye dominance can also change with head position (i.e., rotation of the head can change the eye dominance) or rotation of the torso. When we couple eye dominance with hand dominance, the number of variables that can change and influence the experiential equation of palpation increases exponentially. If we add in that the body placement of the practitioner in relationship to the patient also plays a role in influencing palpation, the equation gets even more complex. This leads to these questions: If each of these different approaches can affect interexaminer reliability, are any of the schools or governing bodies considering and/or teaching this? Are there any research studies that take this into account when examining the results?

If protocol treatment methods are used for most studies for the purpose of reproducibility, is it any wonder why the results don't show consistency, given the numerous variables not accounted for in the examining and testing phases? To get clearer answers would take a study designed to remove the practitioners' biases before the testing begins. It begs the question of whether evidence-based testing is even applicable or fair for osteopathic treatment outcomes.

It would be similar to having a study on a single drug's efficacy that starts with each patient taking a pile of pills daily (only a few of which have been labeled) and expecting good results on the one studied drug. Yet, this is exactly what seems to be happening within osteopathy's evidence-based research.

During courses taught by Osteopathic Vision, LLC, the instructors spend one-on-one time with each practitioner in a small three- or four-person group to sort out their biases. The instructors talk about the findings and lessons mentioned above and then teach and test each of the participants. The participants each gain insight on their personal approach to diagnosis and treatment. Instructors encourage the group to check each other's findings to help integrate less biased methods. This seems to significantly reduce, but not eliminate, the differences in findings between practitioners in courses. It would be interesting to see what would happen if this same instruction were conducted early in every osteopath's education and career.

Another confounding factor in interexaminer reliability is layer palpation—being able to identify exactly what tissue the practitioner is feeling. During my own training, my class learned how to palpate bone, muscles, and fascia as first- and second-year students. This seemed as if it was enough to get the job done, until, as undergraduate fellows, a group of three of us felt something that we had never felt before: a new type/layer of tissue. It took more than six months before we met someone who could give a name to what we felt (periosteum). Over the years, in collaboration with other practitioners, each of us has added layers to our palpation: fluid, fascia, bone, ligament, blood vessels, organs, etc. This small group feels fairly adept at being able to identify the layer each can now palpate. This is something that was not taught directly in our undergraduate or postgraduate educations. Courses on layer palpation are not routine. Would such a course aid in improving interexaminer reliability?

Stiles often tells stories of his mentors in heated arguments disagreeing on what each person was feeling. He learned that for two practitioners to communicate effectively, they first had to define how they described what they were feeling and then how they interpreted those findings. This often led to their realizing that they were arguing about the same layer, dysfunction, or landmark, but using different words to describe it. Teaching through stories, Stiles has left an impression on his students and led many osteopaths to examine carefully how others palpate and describe what they feel. This has helped many of Stiles's students in their individual teaching practices.

The story of Stiles and Huff related above resulted in two masters finding two different key lesions, with the only discovered difference being the layer in which they were searching. Without the group's questions, this difference in their layer of palpation may never have been discovered. Is it any wonder that interexaminer reliability is so poor? There are multiple variables that may differ between practitioners and their treatments. A single change cannot account for all other variables. Is it any wonder osteopaths have such a hard time "proving" osteopathy to the modern medical world when assessment, diagnosis, and treatment are so varied? Modern medicine wants one-size-fits-most treatments, whereas osteopathy may always remain a bespoken treatment for every patient at every visit.

As you study the Long Lever Technique and osteopathy, do you know your biases? Have you worked at learning and removing your own confounding factors? How is your own layer palpation? Can you palpate the fascial and ligamentous layers? Can you discriminate between the two, and can you lock out one and not the other (as Stiles and Huff were doing above)? To do so involves Fryette's laws, but that is not the only thing you need to know how to apply. Can you then locate the primary respiratory mechanism and turn on its potency in the focused area being treated? These are a few of the basic skills that improve mastery of this work but are likely only a small subset of the quanta of the osteopathy you bring to your patients' healing. Does working on this self-awareness increase your treatment outcomes or speed the process along? Here's to continued learning about ourselves and our patients and encouragement to dig on!

Establishing a Medical Practice Where the Long Lever Technique Can Help You Thrive

FRANCOIS L. CYR, MBA

Congratulations on learning the Long Lever Technique! Applying this treatment modality in practice will provide important and immediate benefits to your patients and your medical practice. The Long Lever Technique can help increase efficiency, as well as increase revenue.

I have managed a private osteopathic medical practice for more than fifteen years and have counseled many doctors, residents, and medical students on how to best establish and operate a private osteopathic medical practice. In that role, I am constantly amazed and excited to hear how many of these practitioners desire to have an independent, private medical practice in which to provide osteopathic manipulation for their patients.

A common concern is that doctors often have neither knowledge nor training in business to understand how to manage a medical practice. Physicians are highly educated, capable individuals who continually study and review large amounts of information to maintain the knowledge and skills necessary to be successful. So then, when do they have time to learn the *business* of medicine? Doctors are not trained to run businesses, but to provide specialized care to those in need. The fact is, many are averse to discuss the business of medicine, as they neither understand nor even care to know it.

Fortunately, there are many resources available to assist doctors to learn both practice management and best clinical practices. Among these resources are medical associations, small business development agencies, and companies that provide medical practice support. There are also numerous informative publications, websites, and videos available.

Two fundamental points to be aware of when discussing medicine and business:

1. Doctors providing osteopathic manipulative services are sorely needed. The services they provide are desired by many, even if they do not know it yet. Physicians

who practice osteopathic manipulation, including the Long Lever Technique, offer invaluable services that greatly benefit the health of patients and the vitality of clinical practices.

2. To be successful, it is imperative to know the business side of clinical practice. Whether physicians work for themselves, as employees in a group or managed care practice, or in academia, they must become knowledgeable about how to properly evaluate and bill for the medical services they provide and about how these services impact the total income of their practices. *It all affects the bottom line.*

According to a 2016 article written by David Squires and David Blumenthal, MD, "Between 1983 and 2014, the percentage of physicians practicing alone fell from 41% to 17%."[3] The number of private practice physicians in the United States has been declining for years. This is due to a number of factors, but it suffices to say that doctors in private practice are a minority. Some private practice physicians believe this works in their favor, allowing them to position themselves in unique niches in the marketplace. Private practice allows for development of individual and distinct styles of practice, often without undo competition.

Today, most physicians work for hospitals or group practices. They are provided a salary, benefits, and a retirement plan. This can be attractive, and there are benefits, but there are also drawbacks. An important factor to note is that employed physicians have a limited ability to truly manage their clinical work. They are limited by their scope of practice, where they practice, patient loads, and the amount of independence they have in providing which services to their patients. Limits are set by the system or group, and each group or system has a bureaucracy to be navigated in order to be successful.

The private practice model is quite simple by comparison. The physician makes all of the decisions and can practice how he or she chooses. Decisions, such as how big to grow or how small to stay, how much to spend, and how much to take home, are completely up to the clinician. Most importantly, medical decision making is completely independent and autonomous. Additionally, private practice physicians possess total and complete control over their practices: where, when, what, and how they practice, as well as how much to charge which patients for services.

It has been my experience, based on those with whom I have met, that many osteopaths who work in a group or hospital setting, and who also provide osteopathic manipulation, are often frustrated. They may be limited in how and when they can offer osteopathic manipulative treatment or are plainly told that osteopathic manipulation is not to be offered by their practices. Others are equally frustrated by billing departments or staff who do not know how to properly bill and collect for their services, thus affecting the calculation of clinical productivity and, subsequently, individual income.

---

[3] Squires, D., & Blumenthal, D. (May 2016). "Do small physician practices have a future?" Commonwealth Fund. www.commonwealthfund.org/blog/2016/do-small-physician-practices-have-future.

Private practice physicians have few of these challenges. These physicians choose when and how to provide services to which patients and how to charge for those services, especially if they are fee-for-service or cash practices that do not accept direct insurance payments. This is the simplest model to offer and deliver osteopathic manipulative services. With the intricacies and stylistic differences between osteopaths in how they treat and the services they provide, private practice physicians are in the best position to decide which of their services are in the best interests of their patients and their practices.

So, how does the Long Lever Technique work in practice? The Long Lever Technique can be incorporated into any type of practice or practice setting. Generally, visits for osteopathic manipulative medicine average 30 minutes or more, limiting the number of patients who may be seen in a given hour or day. Those who utilize direct techniques, such as HVLA, often have shorter visits but may also provide less long-term relief for their patients. The solution? The Long Lever Technique. This can increase efficiency by producing faster and longer-lasting benefits in treatment. The physician utilizing the Long Lever Technique may see an increase in both the number of patients who benefit long term, as well as the ability to do more in less time. This directly helps both patients and doctors by minimizing the length of patient visits while increasing the positive results from osteopathic treatment.

Is it better to be an employee or to have a private practice? Some physicians believe they will always be employed and cannot truly consider the possibility of working in a private osteopathic practice. It is true that certain clinical specialties require the resources and services that only a hospital can provide. However, for many physicians they can "have their cake and eat it too." It is possible to be employed and also have an independent clinical practice providing osteopathic manipulation to patients. There may be some geographical and legal limits that come into play as physicians explore how and where to open their practices, but most often, these limitations can be easily overcome.

There are many strategies on how to best start a practice, regardless of whether a physician is newly graduated or has been in practice for years. The key is to develop a plan on how best to incorporate osteopathic manipulation and the Long Lever Technique into their practices. It is also very important to get advice and counsel to develop a plan, whether expanding an existing private practice or opening a new private practice. There are numerous resources available to help physicians: the internet; state, county, and city governments; the Small Business Administration; and the local chamber of commerce all have helpful information and materials for anyone who is interested in starting their own business. Additional resources are available from medical associations on best practices and on opening and managing a private medical practice.

Afterword

D r. Richard Huff grew up in Kirksville, Missouri, where he was treated by the local osteopathic physicians trained at what was then Kirksville College of Osteopathic Medicine. By the time I joined him in practice as we set up a residency training program in neuromusculoskeletal medicine at Mercy Health Partners in Muskegon, Michigan, he had been developing his approach to OMT for more than three decades.

As we developed the residency program, Dr. Huff told me he saw himself more as a practitioner than a teacher. I was surprised: here was a man who was approaching an age to retire a second time but had never stopped being a student. He still read from a broad variety of sources and disciplines in his effort to greater understand the care of his patients. He kept exploring new ideas, experimenting with new techniques, and refining his approach; in his words, he kept "reinventing" himself.

Doctors in the West Michigan community regularly referred to him the "difficult" patients: those with chronic pain or fatigue, difficult-to-manage headaches, myofascial pain or fibromyalgia, temporomandibular joint dysfunction, failed back syndrome, nonsurgical abdominal pain, or other difficult-to-explain symptoms. Dr. Huff welcomed these cases both as a challenge and, more importantly, because he believed he could help.

While Dr. Huff was a lifelong learner, these "difficult" patient cases benefited also from the many interactions Dr. Huff had with fellow osteopaths. From his training in Kirksville to a yearlong neuroanatomy fellowship (alongside Jim Jealous, DO, who was the anatomy fellow), to impromptu workshops with senior osteopaths (including Robert Fulford, DO, FCA) at the Annual Convocation of the American Academy of Osteopathy, Dr. Huff thrived on the shared pursuit of better techniques and better outcomes for patients. Importantly, Dr. Huff often noted the patients themselves contributed to the knowledge that in turn helped other patients and, ultimately, resulted in the Long Lever Technique, a well-tolerated and effective way to help restore function.

In my position alongside Dr. Huff training future osteopaths, I enjoyed hearing residents discuss their craft and passion. Notably, early residents articulated OMT ideas differently than later residents; I think this is the result of Dr. Huff's continuous learning and desire to find more new, effective techniques for full function. The later residents fluently discussed and used the concepts outlined in this *Long Lever Techniques* manual. I think this manual represents the best compilation of explanations and descriptions of what Dr. Huff did with his hands to optimize function of each patient's self-healing, self-regulating mechanism.

I still reflect on Dr. Huff's perception of himself as a student more than a teacher. I think his continuous experimenting and learning placed him firmly in the role of student even when he was an experienced OMT practitioner. I suspect this mode of lifelong ideation helped him connect with students who were for the first time attempting to convert lectures on palpation into, literally, hands-on practice. Students frequently mimic techniques they think the teacher is demonstrating, but in OMT this demonstration-to-practice process may not result in the student experiencing the same palpatory experience as the teacher. When the student shifts from mimicry of motions and positions to engaging in a dialogue with a patient's tissues, the student begins to understand and learn from the natural laws that govern the health and life of the body.

I also reflect on Dr. Huff's use of the primary respiratory mechanism as a diagnostic guide and as a force for the correction of the abnormal toward the normal. When an experienced OMT practitioner observes the primary respiratory mechanism for diagnosis and treatment, the process may look easy from the outside. But this process takes practice; in all manner of osteopathic manipulation, the ability to listen to the "hum of the engine of life" to interpret accurately the cause of some "rough idling," identify a disturbance in how "power is transmitted," or detect a vibration that may eventually lead to excessive "wear and failure" is an acquired skill necessary both for accurate diagnosis and for appropriate treatment.

The more subtle practice of close listening and palpation is a hallmark of effective OMT. As A.T. Still articulated about a physician, "He must not be like a blacksmith, only able to hit large bones and muscles with a heavy hammer, but he must be able to use the most delicate instruments of the silversmith in adjusting the deranged, displaced bones, nerves, muscles, and remove all obstructions, and thereby restore the machinery of life to its normal movement. To do this is to be an osteopath."[4] In this manual, Drs. Huff and Nourani have collected information on and explained the use of Long Lever Techniques to enable physicians to work with this approach and feel the effectiveness of it with their own patients and hands. For some physicians, this manual may be validation for phenomena they have observed but have not found language to describe. For other physicians, this manual may shift their treatment paradigm. But for all physicians, I hope this manual enables familiarity with another method to exercise the "delicate instruments of the silversmith" as we physicians work to restore the machinery of life.

Michael Carnes, DO, FAAO

Associate Professor, Osteopathic Principles and Practice

University of Pikeville–Kentucky College of Osteopathic Medicine

---

[4] Still, A.T. (1908). *Autobiography of A.T. Still,* rev. ed. Kirksville, MO: A.T. Still.Chapter XXIV, p. 290.

Acknowledgments by Content Editors

Much gratitude is owed to Bobby Nourani, DO, FAAO, for capturing in writing the thoughts and techniques of Richard Huff, DO, a wonderful osteopathic leader and teacher. Dr. Huff often felt limited by the words available to explain his approach to OMT. I believe one of Dr. Nourani's real successes in this LLT manual is to capture Dr. Huff's thoughts and perceptions rather than simply explaining the work he was doing.

I had the privilege of learning from Dr. Huff during my NMM/OMM residency at Mercy Health Partners in Muskegon, Michigan. His primary teaching method was hand-over-hand. I distinctly remember upon finding a restricted region to be addressed that he would place his large hand over mine, quickly localize all the planes of an appropriate barrier, and press his fingers down on mine, while I would feel nothing but the pressure of his hand. While waiting for the inherent forces to do their work, he would note when rotation began to improve, then flexion/extension, until finally observing the integration above and below the segment. Despite this direct guidance, it took several years for me to feel and understand the true application of the LLT with its use of localization at the barrier and the power of inherent forces.

I now have students' hands under my hands. I describe the setup at the barrier, the inherent forces, and the release. As a teacher, I continue to appreciate the difficulty in describing palpatory nuances so as not to interfere with the experiential learning of the student.

This manual is an excellent starting point to better understand inherent forces in augmenting treatment for all levels of training. I am grateful for the work Drs. Nourani, Carnes, and others have done to succinctly describe Dr. Huff's love and legacy.

Kate Heineman, DO

Richard Huff, DO, was most influential in developing my sense of man-as-machine in the biomechanical model of osteopathy. His ongoing pursuit of practical applications for anatomical knowledge inspired me to dig deeper into the possibilities osteopathic physicians can accomplish with hands and minds working in both artistic and scientific concert.

Dr. Huff's LLT has proved to be not only an effective but also an efficient means to address biomechanical restrictions. LLT makes sense to my patients. They can feel the fascial leverage at the site of their dysfunction, are aware of the pseudo-barriers, and can feel a barrier releasing. These techniques have earned their place in my preferred style of osteopathic treatments.

Bobby Nourani was a close colleague in training, and I have always appreciated his attention to detail and subtlety. In his hands the LLT is not an instrument of force but rather one of precision. This focus on precision is one of Dr. Huff's fundamental truths that I think will become clear to osteopathic students and physicians using these techniques.

Benjamin J. Visger, DO

Taking the teachings of his mentor and friend, Richard Huff, DO, Dr. Nourani has beautifully organized and presented the life's work of a master of osteopathic manipulation so that it might not be lost to future generations of healers. To me, this is their greatest achievement. Whether this treatment style resonates with the reader and becomes a keystone in the approach to patient treatment is not nearly as important as having the information and the clear explanation of its application from the one who developed the modality as seen through the eyes of one who successfully learned to utilize its principles.

This manual provides Dr. Huff's explanation of what he did and why he did it that way and shows in a step-by-step manner how to set up and perform what he did. As with any good technique manual, Dr. Nourani clearly and simply shows where to stand and what to hold, and then explains how to get the primary respiratory force to actualize the treatment. Dr. Huff's perspective provides insight into how and why he came to develop this treatment form, something most technique manuals lack. I was taught by my mentor to study the masters, what they did, and how they performed it, but to be careful in listening to their explanations of their craft, because they were often wrong. Still, hearing the ideas in their own words, and more than just a technical description, can personalize the action so that the intent of treatment may also be realized. Principles are then internalized, and mastery is then only a matter of practice. It is a privilege to be a part of developing such a work.

William P. Powell, DO

Acknowledgments

This manual could not have been created without the years of experience, hard work, teachings, and patience of Richard Huff, DO. Many have asked him to write up his techniques. I am grateful that he entrusted me with documentation and creative organization to present his teachings in this manual. It is an honor to have been asked to deliver this valuable treatment tool to the world of osteopathy.

Dr. Huff told me, "I can show you everything I know in two weeks." Though I believed him, I knew it would take longer to effectively apply his teachings with any confidence and mastery, with consistent results. The more I have focused on the theory, rather than the techniques, the faster my patients have improved.

Authoring this text was initially encouraged by Michael Carnes, DO. Under his directorship during my Neuromusculoskeletal Medicine Plus One year, he instilled the confidence in me to produce this manual. His repeated support, from conceptualization through the publication of this manual, was nothing short of inspiring.

A special thanks to the team members at Mercy Health Partners who directly assisted in creating the *Long Lever Techniques* manual:

Richard Huff, DO	Shannon Crout, DO	Sheri Hull, DO
Michael Carnes, DO	Ben Visger, DO	Zach Musgrave, DO
Paul Dyball, DO	Michelle Visger	Katje Musgrave, DO
Amelia Bueche, DO	Stella Emsellem, DO	
Kate Heineman, DO	Victoria Chang, DO	

I appreciate Dr. Visger's review and edits. Our countless hours teasing out the descriptions to better inform the reader have yielded this product, which we are proud to say represents a glimpse of the brilliance Dr. Huff imparted on us. Many thanks to Dr. Heineman's skillful content edits of Dr. Huff's drafts. Her ability to maintain Dr. Huff's voice and convey his message to the reader are much appreciated. A warm thank you to the additional reviewers: Bill Powell, DO; Kelli Sharp, DPT; Lilian Au, ND, MPH; Susan Yoo-Lee; Elaine Rosenberg; Brett Huff; and Christopher Muller.

Thank you, Bill Kuchera, DO, FAAO, Dist., for the medical illustrations you created. What a joy to create educational art from our combined mental visions! Thank you to photographer and graphics editor Jim Keating. Your skillful and artistic enhancement resulted in clarity of images to visually relay detailed descriptions. Without your dedication and continued support, completion of this project would not have been possible.

I want to thank all of my mentors and teachers who have guided me to be the physician I am today. You have guided me toward my optimal potential and consistently nourished my continuous growth as a physician. In order of when you first cultivated me with your osteopathic wisdom:

Arash Jacob, DO

Brett Thomas, DO

Viola Frymann, DO

Mary Anne Morelli, DO

Sean Centers, DO

Charlie Beck, DO

Deborah Heath, DO

Peter Springall, PhD

Bill Petras, DO

2004–2008 AZCOM

Bill Devine, DO

Steve Davidson, DO

Lori Kemper, DO

Richard Dobrusin, DO

Barry Malina, DO

Anna Svircev, DO

Eric Dolgin, DO

Paul Dart, MD

Darick Nordstrom, DDS

Damon Whitfield, DO

Sean Tsai, DO

Paul Hume, ND, DO

Philippe Druelle, DO

Laura Rampil, DO

Thomas Crow, DO

Laura Griffin, DO

Jaimee Lippert, DO

Elizabeth Kronlage, DO

Hugh Ettlinger, DO

Eliott Blackman, DO

Ed Stiles, DO

Josh Dalton, DO

Derek Jones, DO

Bill Powell, DO

Bruno Chikly, MD, DO

Luna Leyva, MD

Cynthia Kodama, DO

Hovsep Babayan, DO

Hieu Nguyen, DO

Eric Lin, DO

Theresa Cyr, DO

Francois Cyr, MBA

Richard Huff, DO

Michael Carnes, DO

Michael Seffinger, DO

Paul Dyball, DO

Amelia Bueche, DO

Ali Carine, DO

Tudor Marinescu, MD

Andrew Kochan, MD

Ben Bullington, MD

Jeff Ericksen, MD

Jeff Patterson, DO

Jorge Moreno, DO

David Holt, DO

Jerry Sparby

Rick Owens, MD

David Wang, DO

Ali Safayan, MD

John Sarcar, MD

Joe Helms, MD

Howard Rosen, MD

Mary Doherty

Paul Johnson, DO

David Rabago, MD

Marty Gallagher, MD, DC

Bruce Flagg, DO

Ken Lossing, DO

Carrie Carda, MD

Michael Kuchera, DO

Rachel Brooks, MD

Becki Giusti, DO

John Hughes, DO

Lilia Gorodinsky, DO

and to all those to come,
Thank You.

Bobby Nourani, DO, FAAO

Index

About the Authors

RICHARD HUFF, DO (1943–2019), synthesized the Long Lever Technique concept as a fusion of A.T. Still's and W.G. Sutherland's principles for effective and time-efficient treatment. Dr. Huff was an avid learner, well-respected clinician, and invaluable instructor of manual medicine. He was a devoted leader in the osteopathic community and founded the Neuromusculoskeletal Medicine residency program in West Michigan. The osteopathic legacy of Richard Huff, DO, is presented in this manual.

BOBBY NOURANI, DO, FAAO, is an expert in the area of integrative musculoskeletal pain medicine. His clinical, academic, and research contributions support the use of treatment approaches that are well received by patients and peers. Dr. Nourani is associate professor in the Department of Neuromusculoskeletal Medicine/Osteopathic Manipulative Medicine (NMM/OMM) at the College of Osteopathic Medicine of the Pacific, Western University of Health Sciences. His past positions include the program director of Osteopathic Curriculum and Instruction at the University of Wisconsin and medical director of the Inpatient Integrative Health Consult Service at the University of California–Irvine. He is board certified in Neuromusculoskeletal Medicine as well as Family Medicine & Osteopathic Manipulative Treatment and holds a certificate of added qualifications in Pain Medicine. He advanced and expanded the Long Lever Techniques as taught by his mentor, Dr. Huff, and utilizes them in his teaching and practice.

About North Atlantic Books

North Atlantic Books (NAB) is a 501(c)(3) nonprofit publisher committed to a bold exploration of the relationships between mind, body, spirit, culture, and nature. Founded in 1974, NAB aims to nurture a holistic view of the arts, sciences, humanities, and healing. To make a donation or to learn more about our books, authors, events, and newsletter, please visit www.northatlanticbooks.com.

01 14